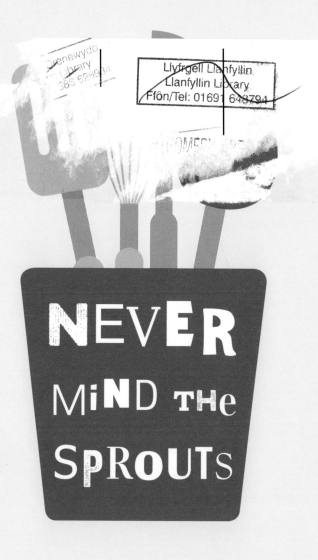

NEVER
MiND THe
SPROUTs

NEVER MIND THE SPROUTS

Vie Books is an imprint of Summersdale Publishers Ltd

Summersdale Publishers Ltd
46 West Street
Chichester
West Sussex
PO19 1RP
UK

www.summersdale.com

Printed and bound in the Czech Republic

ISBN: 978-1-84953-569-4

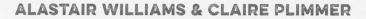

ALASTAIR WILLIAMS & CLAIRE PLIMMER

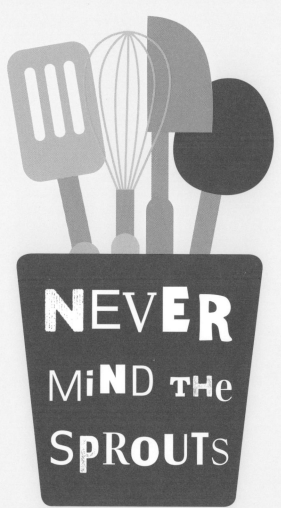

NEVER MiND THe SpROUTs

SIMPLE AND EASY RECIPES THAT
ALL THE FAMILY WILL ENJOY...
ESPECIALLY FUSSY EATERS

This book is dedicated to
Kitty, Freddie, Elizabeth and Piers,
with all our love

CONTENTS

INTRODUCTION

You may have picked up this book because you would love your child to be a 'good' eater – not a 'fussy' eater – a child who's consuming a nutritious and balanced diet. It's only natural.

From the moment we become parents, it seems that we are programmed to worry and one of our key concerns is to make sure our child eats well so that he or she grows and develops healthily. The worry that your child has not put on those requisite ounces during their formative weeks is the start point of a concern that can gather momentum as milk feeds switch to the weaning process and beyond.

There is so much advice available to parents with regard to how best to nourish a child, and whole industries have been established around this topic. You may still be haunted by the guilt that during the weaning process you didn't have the time (or maybe the inclination) to steam, purée and pack ice cube trays full of organic vegetables in order to prepare baby-sized chunks of frozen goodness. And even if you did go through the trials of such preparation, all of your hard work and effort may have been thwarted when your child took one baby spoonful of the warmed-up goo only to projectile spit it out at you. Maybe things didn't get any better for you as they moved on to finger food, preferring a strict diet of breadsticks against any sniff of a carrot baton.

It could be that the transition to full meals saw no further joy. At a time when we know it's crucial for our child's health that they eat the correct amount of vitamins, minerals, proteins and starches, your child won't touch anything green and turns their nose up at any kind of protein. Your friends' children appear to be eating really well, yet all your child wants to munch on is jam sandwiches.

If this sounds all too familiar fear not; you are not alone. Many parents encounter these kinds of scenarios and, try as you might to create a model eater, mealtime battles are experienced by what seems to be the vast majority of us. If you have a child who does not clap their hands in delight when you serve up a 'good for you' dish, don't beat yourself up, there will usually be a way to find something nourishing that they'll like, and that something could be a simple dish of home-made fish fingers and peas. We won't guarantee that your child will suddenly eat everything but, with a little help from this book, there can be light at the end of the tunnel.

There are usually ways to get through eating barriers and one of the best places to start is for you to stop being stressed about it. Tastes can be developed and a more varied diet is achievable.

As authors, we are not parenting or nutritional experts; we are parents with experience of dealing with difficult eaters. This book is designed to give some pointers on ways you can try to change poor eating habits or break down the barriers that may have been formed against eating, such as decisions not to eat certain foods that have been made based on a bad eating experience. It also provides you with a one-stop shop of ideas and recipes for simple meals and snacks, all delivered with straight-forward preparation instructions.

Some of the recipes within this book are very basic and not always true to some of the original recipes that you might know and trust – they simply offer a start point that can be embellished as your child's tastes develop.

That said, each recipe in this book is based on simple yet nutritious ingredients that are easy to prepare for busy parents. Alongside some recipes to cook, we've included some no-cook ideas – raw food can have greater health benefits than cooked.

You'll soon discover that not only can food become a great adventure that children will want to join you on, but you could save money by preparing things from scratch.

As part of the research for this book we questioned close to 200 parents and their children to find out what their best and worst foods are, why they like or hate things and what made them change their minds about certain foods. We asked parents what issues they faced with fussy eaters and garnered their opinions about what worked or didn't work for them in their attempts to persuade children to eat. From the evidence collected, one key conclusion can be drawn: tastes do develop and change as children grow older, so it's worth persevering with your child in your quest to change their eating habits. The results of the questionnaire are documented within the book, and useful comments made by parents are sprinkled throughout. Thank you to all of you who helped us with this survey.

We hope that you'll find some quick-win suggestions here, as well as some recipes that will turn into family favourites.

THE BASICS

Common sense

The recipes in this book are designed with simplicity in mind, both in terms of equipment and cooking skills required. Before you try any recipe, read it through first to make sure you have all the ingredients and equipment as well as the time to prepare it. One handy piece of kit to have in the kitchen if you have a fussy eater is a blender (either the handheld variety or the stand alone) as many of the recipes have the option of blitzing ingredients to make them more palatable for your child.

Conversion chart

The recipes in this book are given in metric measurements, but many small amounts are measured in terms of spoons.

The following abbreviations are used:

tbsp = tablespoon

tsp = teaspoon

1 tbsp = 25 g of… syrup, jam, honey, etc.

2 tbsp = 25 g of… butter, sugar

3 tbsp = 25 g of… cornflour, cocoa, custard powder, flour

4 tbsp = 25 g of… grated cheese, porridge oats

All spoon measures refer to level spoons, not heaped.

In all recipes the oven should be heated to the temperature stated prior to cooking to allow it to warm up. Ovens may vary but as a rule of thumb, Celsius is roughly half the Fahrenheit temperature.

Set fan-assisted ovens 25 degrees Celsius (approximately 50 degrees Fahrenheit) lower than others or reduce the cooking time by 10 minutes for every hour of cooking time.

Advice on freezing

Basic advice for freezer storage time:

Fruits (6 months); vegetables (6 months); fish (10 weeks); red meat and chicken (10 weeks).

Nutritional advice

It can be tempting to turn to ready-meals, especially when we're pressured by time or maybe lack confidence in the kitchen, but remember there is nothing more delicious or healthier than home-cooked meals. We often forget in our quest for convenience that processed food is full of hidden fats, sugars and salt.

Our recipes are not a blueprint for the perfect diet; they are simply suggestions to give you options to try. We will not be discussing the 'whys and wherefores' of organic foods in this book (we'll leave you to make that call) but all we'll say is, where possible, fresh is best. Eating fresh fruit and vegetables when they are in season locally makes a lot of sense as they are at their best, and cheapest.

We've provided some basic information to help you make your choices about what to prepare for your child.

Foods are categorised into seven main nutrients: protein, carbohydrate, sugars, fat, saturates (saturated fat), fibre and salt. An individual's nutritional requirements can vary with gender, weight, activity levels and age. GDAs (Guided Daily Amounts) are guidelines for an average person of a healthy weight (i.e. someone who is not intending to lose or gain weight) and an average level of activity. It is a good idea to speak to a doctor or registered dietician if you have specific concerns about diet or weight management.

Average daily kcal requirements for younger children

	Babies 7–12 months	Toddlers aged 1–3	Pre-school children	Children aged 5–10
Boys	545–690	1,230	1,715	1,800
Girls	515–645	1,165	1,545	1,750

(source of data: www.kidsandnutrition.co.uk)

Proteins

The word protein derives from the Greek word meaning 'of first importance', and that is exactly what they are. Proteins are necessary for bodily development and for repairs to damaged cells.

Proteins are typically found in the following foods:

- meat, poultry, and fish;
- eggs;
- legumes (beans and peas);
- tofu;
- soya products;
- grains, nuts and seeds;
- milk and milk products (cheese, yoghurts);
- some vegetables and some fruits (provide only small amounts of protein relative to other sources).

Carbohydrates

These are the providers of energy. Carbohydrates are predominantly divided into two groups, simple and complex carbohydrates.

Simple carbohydrates contribute very little in the way of other nutrients. They are also often high in calories and are found in the following foods:

- fructose or fruit sugar and glucose;
- table sugar;
- fizzy drinks;
- sweets.

Complex carbohydrates are better for you than simple carbohydrates because they tend to be found in plant-based foods where other vital nutrients are present, such as fibre and vitamins. They are found in the following foods:

- cereal and grain (bread, flour, pasta); rice;
- some fruit and vegetables (potatoes, carrots, root vegetables);
- pulses (beans and lentils).

Fats

These provide energy for the body, but they take longer to digest than carbohydrates. This means they are useful for storing energy. Fats are loosely divided into unsaturated and saturated fats, and are best told apart by their consistency: saturated fats are solid at room temperature, whilst unsaturated fats remain liquid at room temperature. Saturated fat should be consumed in moderation. Unsaturated fat, in moderation, is good for you, helping the body to absorb nutrients and providing energy.

Saturated fats are found in:

- all animal fats (e.g. milk fat, lard);
- palm oil;
- coconut oil;
- cocoa fat;
- hydrogenated vegetable oil.

Unsaturated fats are found in:

- vegetable fats;
- sunflower oil;
- olives and olive oil;
- peanut oil;
- maize or corn oil;
- soybeans;
- avocados;
- lean meat;
- fish.

Fibre

Also known as roughage, this is vital if you want to have a healthy functioning digestive system and avoid constipation.

Fibre is found in the following foods:

- beans;
- wholegrain/wholemeal (bread, pasta, rice);
- nuts;
- jacket potato;
- dried fruit;
- cereal/bran;
- porridge;
- fruit and vegetables.

Vitamins

Vitamins are essential nutrients that your body needs in small amounts to work properly.

Vitamin A: is present in dairy products such as cheese, eggs and milk; in green vegetables, fish and liver.

Vitamin B: is made up of more than 10 different vitamins, which are found in wholegrain cereals, liver, yeast, lean meat, beans, peas and nuts.

Vitamin C: is present in citrus fruits such as lemons and oranges, in blackcurrants and fresh vegetables.

Vitamin D: is present in milk, butter, cheese, fish and liver.

Vitamin E: is found in vegetables such as avocados, tomatoes, spinach and watercress; blackberries, mangoes, nuts, wholegrains, olive oil, mackerel and salmon.

Vitamin K: is found in green vegetables and wholegrain cereals.

Minerals

There are three main minerals: iron, calcium and iodine. Other minerals are phosphates, potassium, magnesium and sodium.

Iron: is found in liver, red meat, dried herbs, seeds and dark leafy vegetables.

Calcium: is found in dairy products such as milk, butter and cheese; tofu and soya products and leafy green vegetables.

Iodine: is found in fish, milk, yoghurt and seaweed.

Salt

The general advice on salt is to avoid it, and not to add it to food unnecessarily. However, if you're of the opinion that salt enhances the flavour of a dish and you cannot cook without it, try to be as sparing as possible. Our recipes indicate where salt could be added if you want to use it but, equally, the recipes work without it. The choice is yours.

HOW TO GET STARTED

HABITS

Eating habits and tastes tend to be formed in early childhood. If you are lucky, your child will sail through the early years munching on all sorts of things with no problems but, for many of us, fussy eating habits in our children develop soon after weaning. For others, a toddler might seem perfectly content eating whatever is put in front of them only to start being picky as they become able to articulate their choices.

Until your child's taste buds develop, they'll most likely prefer bland food against spicy or complex taste combinations – if you're having trouble finding flavours that your child would like, you may have to revert to a simpler menu and range of flavours to jump start their eating. Sometimes going back to basics will be your way of happening upon dishes that even the fussiest of eaters will enjoy.

FAMILIARISATION

Some children develop a fear of eating. One good way of trying to overcome any such phobia is to re-familiarise your child with the normality of food and eating, which is a chance for you to spend time together with food.

We suggest that you get your children to join in with a variety of food-related activities, from helping you with the shopping to assisting with the cooking too, you could even have a go at growing your ingredients together – the more familiar they are with foodstuffs the better. Getting them involved is not only a great way of passing on food knowledge but it helps them to feel at one with what they're eating.

SOCIALISATION

Once you've prepared a meal, sitting down together to eat can be an important aspect of family life. Mealtimes are a simple yet effective way of strengthening bonds within the family, by not only bringing you together to share food, but providing an opportunity for you to talk to each other without distractions. Finding that one meal that everyone can enjoy together in this way is a real boon (not to mention a blessing for the chef of the house).

There's a connotation between home-cooked food and comfort. The pleasure derived from preparing a meal for your loved ones and watching them eat and enjoy your food cannot be questioned.

TOP TIPS

The following pointers will help you out in your quest to turn your child into a 'good eater' but if in doubt, the key is to remember that if you are struggling you are not alone, and to try not to beat yourself up about it:

Look at the positives
- Make a list of all the things your child does eat, you might just be surprised.

Try not to force the issue
- If you insist that a child does something, you are bound to confront their iron will and, where food is concerned, they can become accomplished at firmly refusing to eat.

- If you present food with the message: 'eat it, it's good for you', your child will simply hear, 'Yuck, that's what you said when you tried to make me eat sprouts' and the automatic response will be resistance.

- Try to get your child to take responsibility for their eating. A good way to start is by placing food in the middle of the table at mealtimes and asking your child to serve themselves. You'll be surprised at the positive results this small action can have.

Keep it simple

- It's quite normal for children to want to be able to identify the food they are eating. Hiding things in a sauce can be off-putting and can lead to your child spending the whole mealtime picking 'bits' out. If you find that your child prefers to see clearly what's in their food, don't be afraid to go along with this desire as you try to get them to eat and try new foods.

- A dish containing just a few elements can seem more manageable for a child than a feast of different things to taste. Some children don't like the different elements of the dish they're eating to be touching each other; if this is the case, simply arrange food in a way that means your child is happy to eat it.

We eat with all of our senses, not just taste

- The way things are presented can be a deal-breaker, too much on a plate can be a complete turn-off, especially to a child.

- Persevere with different textures – anecdotal impressions gleaned from our food survey clearly indicate that texture is a key driver in a child's like or dislike of a food. It's tempting to purée stuff because that's what very young children are brought up on so it's what they are used to but, the longer you keep to purées, the more difficult it will be to transition to different textures.

- Make food colourful – children are often attracted by the most brightly coloured foods.

Bring some fun into eating, especially for young children

- Turn the plate into a picture – mashed-potato hair, peas for eyes, a carrot nose, a sausage smile…

- Create patterns on the plate to make food look more interesting.

- Try different ways of eating – experiment with finger food (sticky rice balls dipped in sauce), prepare a medieval banquet where it's de rigueur to get mucky with drumsticks, dabble with chopsticks, twizzle spaghetti…

- Turn eating into a game – introduce new tastes with a teaspoon test by laying out a range of foodstuffs on a tray and asking your child to describe the flavours – salty or sweet; sour or fresh, etc.

Less is more

- It might seem basic but remember a child's stomach is smaller than an adult's so it doesn't need as much food. It's worth noting that your stomach is approximately the size of your fist, and most of us eat more than we need.

- Most adults have three meals a day. Children on the other hand can be 'grazers' – only wanting to eat when they're hungry. There are mixed opinions about this issue. If you are happy to let your child graze, just make sure their snacks are healthy but remember, the more consumed in between meals, the smaller the appetite at mealtimes.

- Children's appetites can be unpredictable. Some days they'll pick, other days they'll be ravenous. So long as your child averages out with a decent amount of 'fuel', and they are thriving, don't panic when they have an 'off day' – stubbornness will never win over hunger in the end.

Same old, same old

- Don't panic if your child repeatedly eats the same thing. Children like repetition and are quite happy to eat the same thing over and over no matter how dull it might seem to you.

- It's quite normal for children to be 'scared' of some foods; try to be sensitive to this when you introduce something new or unusual. If you want to introduce a new taste or texture, try presenting it alongside some familiar and liked foods.

- Sometimes offering a child a choice of what, or how much to eat can be the road to disaster when a child is fussy (not to mention the nightmare it causes for the person having to prepare three different meals to fit all tastes) – if you use some of the tips above and simply present a dish as a fait accompli at least you don't have to have a battle of negotiation.

If at first you don't succeed

- Remember that it takes at least seven times of tasting something new before reluctant taste buds can really decide whether they're prepared to go along with a new taste.

- If your child doesn't like meat or fish, protein can be found in many other sources such as butter, eggs, milk, cheese, yoghurt, beans and nuts so if you are worried about their protein intake try some vegetarian recipes.

- Every child is different and we cannot claim to provide you with a magic wand to wave but if you give these suggestions a try you may well find a winning solution.

PREPARING FOR TAKE-OFF

Life seems to get busier and busier. Here are a few tips to make life less stressful when it comes to feeding your child or children:

- Get your larder in order. Having standby ingredients can reduce stress for those last minute occasions when you need to prepare something on the hoof. Basics such as: dried foods like pasta and rice; tinned tomatoes and tubes of tomato purée; tins of beans and tuna; jars of pesto and a selection of dried herbs will always come in handy.

- Once you have some larder basics on board you'll be able to buy foodstuffs that are seasonal. As we've discussed, this practice will be kinder on your wallet and the food is likely to be tastier and full of goodness.

- Plan the week's menu if you can: a little forward planning makes cooking much less stressful.

- Cook in advance (e.g. a stew or a casserole) and chill ready-to-eat during the week.

- Stock up your freezer: with a little planning it's easy to cook double quantities of dishes and freeze portions for another day. Home-made frozen meals are a great fall back on busy days when you don't have time to cook from scratch but you're still seeking the comfort of home cooking.

- Have a bash at home-baking instead of buying sweet treats. At least you know what's going into home-made stuff and it's fun for kids if you involve them in the preparation.

On to the recipes… have fun!

NB: the measurements used in each recipe assume four servings.

STAPLES, STOCKS AND SAUCES

BLITZED ONIONS

Many savoury recipes include onions as a key ingredient but onions can be one of those things that fussy eaters cannot abide, especially from a texture point of view. Often, if the onions are hidden, they are happily consumed and a good way of doing this is to purée (blitz) them. To make life easier for you, a useful resource is to prepare a job lot of puréed onions that can be frozen and added to the recipes in this book in place of fresh onions. The amount you choose to make is up to you but here's a rough guideline:

Ingredients:

6 large onions

3 tbsp cooking oil (vegetable or olive)

Peel and chop the onions. Heat the oil in a large frying pan or casserole dish. Gently fry the onions on a low heat until they become translucent, stirring occasionally to make sure they do not stick. It's a good idea to cover the pan or dish with a lid during cooking in order to retain some of the moisture from the onions as this will help with freezing.

Remove the pan or dish from the heat and allow to cool, then blitz the onions until they form a smooth purée. Set aside until completely cooled before transferring the purée into ice cube trays for freezing. Once frozen, decant the onion ice cubes into freezer bags.

The size of your onion ice cubes will dictate the number of cubes you'll need for each recipe, for example, if your ice cube tray is 18 cubes big, and you manage to squeeze a third of your purée into the one tray, you'll have the equivalent of two large onions in a tray so you'll need nine cubes for one large onion, or about six cubes for a medium onion recipe. Remember to keep a note of the equivalent amounts.

TOP TIP

Although it can be a great way of hiding vegetables, don't blitz forever; it won't help in the long run and at some point your child will have to confront joined-up vegetables.

BASIC VEGETABLE STOCK
(makes 1 pint)

Ingredients:

2 medium carrots

1 large onion

1 celery stick

6 black peppercorns

1 dried bay leaf

3 fresh parsley stalks

(A bouquet garni can be used if fresh herbs are not available)

(A range of other vegetables can be used in this stock, broccoli, cabbage, etc.)

Peel and roughly chop the carrots, onion and celery then put all the ingredients into a large pan and cover with water. Bring to the boil. Cover and simmer very gently for 20–30 minutes. Strain into a large bowl and allow to cool.

Use within 3 days or freeze.

This home-made stock is a useful ingredient to have on standby so freezing's a good idea. To do so, reduce the stock by half by boiling vigorously then allow the liquid to cool. Pour into ice cube trays and freeze. When frozen put the cubes into a bag, label it, and when you want to use one, just put in a jug and add boiling water to dissolve the cube.

BASIC CHICKEN STOCK
(makes 1–2 pints)

Ingredients:

1 large carrot

1 large onion

1 celery stick

Bones from a leftover roast chicken carcass

6 black peppercorns

1 dried bay leaf

3 fresh parsley stalks

1 sprig fresh thyme

(A bouquet garni can be used if fresh herbs are not available)

Peel and roughly chop the carrot, onion and celery then put all the ingredients into a large pan and cover with water. Bring to the boil and skim off any scum that has formed. Cover and simmer very gently for 2–3 hours.

Strain into a large bowl and allow to cool. Chill overnight.

Skim off any fat that has formed on the surface. Use within 3 days or freeze.

The home-made nature of this stock gives it real depth of flavour and, like vegetable stock, it's a useful ingredient to have on standby so freezing's a good idea. To do so, reduce the stock by half by boiling vigorously then allow the liquid to cool. Pour into ice cube trays and freeze. When frozen put the cubes into a bag, label it, and when you want to use one, just put in a jug and add boiling water to dissolve the cube.

BASIC WHITE SAUCE

There are lots of variations of white sauces which can be used as a basis for a variety of other sauces. They all start with what's known as a basic roux.

Ingredients:

50 g butter

50 g plain flour

500 ml milk (warmed)

Melt the butter in a small saucepan, but don't let it brown. Then stir in the flour and cook gently for a couple of minutes, stirring continuously to avoid getting any lumps. This is called a roux.

Remove the roux from the heat and add a little of the milk. It has to be added gradually otherwise it will end up being lumpy. Stir in small amounts of milk at a time until a smooth consistency is achieved. When all the milk has been added, return the pan to the heat to thicken.

CHEESE SAUCE

Add 100 g of grated cheese to the white sauce when you return it to the heat. Simmer for 5 minutes or so, then season with salt and pepper to taste. This can be used for cauliflower cheese, lasagne and other pasta dishes.

PARSLEY SAUCE

Add 4 tbsp of chopped fresh parsley to the roux, and salt and pepper to taste, just before serving. This goes especially well with fish dishes.

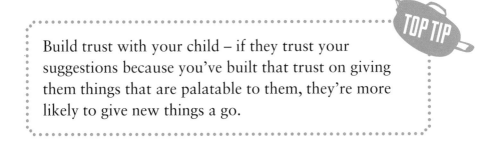

TOP TIP

Build trust with your child – if they trust your suggestions because you've built that trust on giving them things that are palatable to them, they're more likely to give new things a go.

BASIC TOMATO SAUCE

This handy sauce is a staple for pasta dishes and will quickly become a mainstay. You can perk it up in a variety of ways, using different herbs and spices, or adding olives if your child is adventurous. It's best to start off with the most basic version of the sauce to get your child to like it and, once it's become acceptable, you can add to it and try to stop blitzing. The creamy version is often more palatable for children as the cheese takes some of the acidity out of the tomatoes.

Ingredients:

2 cloves of garlic

1 large onion

1 tbsp cooking oil (vegetable or olive)

1 x 400 g can of chopped tomatoes

Seasoning (salt, if desired, and pepper to taste)

Optional additions for the more adventurous (use one of the following):

1 tbsp dried mixed herbs (add alongside the garlic);

A handful of fresh basil (add towards the end of cooking);

1 tsp paprika (add with the tomatoes);

3 tbsp mascarpone cheese (stir in at the end of cooking).

Peel and crush the garlic, and peel and chop the onion. Heat the oil in a large frying pan then gently fry the chopped onion until soft and then add the garlic and fry for a further 3 minutes until translucent. Add the chopped tomatoes and seasoning, bring to the boil, reduce heat and allow to simmer for ten minutes. Blitz the sauce with a hand blender.

PESTO

Children seem to have a love/hate relationship with pesto. It's worth giving it a shot because if your child ends up loving it, it's a quick and easy supper when served with pasta and is a versatile sauce to pep up a variety of dishes. Try spreading it on toast or in a sandwich, drizzle it over chicken or use it as a salad dressing.

Ingredients:

2 cloves of garlic

2 handfuls of fresh basil leaves

50 g pine nuts

3 tbsp Parmesan cheese

125 ml olive oil

Seasoning (salt, if desired, and pepper to taste)

Peel and crush the garlic cloves. Put the garlic, basil leaves and pine nuts in a blender and grind for a few seconds. Grate the cheese then, along with the oil (and seasoning if desired), add to the other ingredients and mix well. If you are a stickler for authenticity, then you should prepare the pesto in a mortar, but blitzing it in a blender is far quicker.

SOUPS

BROCCOLI SOUP
(or green soup as one of our sons calls it)

This wonderfully rich soup has a vibrant colour and a great depth of flavour. If you feel creative, you could invent tales of the special super-power properties found only in this unlikely coloured soup, especially for those who fear any kind of green food.

Ingredients:

1 large onion

2 tbsp cooking oil (vegetable or olive)

750 g broccoli

3 medium potatoes

1.2 l vegetable or chicken stock

Seasoning (salt, if desired, and pepper to taste)

Peel and roughly chop the onion. Heat the oil in a large saucepan on a medium heat. Add the onions and gently fry for 3 minutes until softened then add the broccoli and fry for a further 5 minutes, stirring all the while. Peel and cut the potatoes into medium-sized chunks. Add the potatoes, stock and season to taste. Bring to the boil, then simmer on a lower heat for 20 minutes until the vegetables are soft.

Remove from heat and leave to cool then blitz in a food processor until smooth before returning to the pan to reheat on a low heat for 5 minutes.

Tip: If you want to elaborate on this recipe for those who prefer a more complex flavour, simply chop up some of that leftover blue cheese, Stilton works well, and add it to your own dish when the soup is served.

CARROT SOUP
(with ginger if you can sneak some in!)

This is a gem of a soup, its colour as cheery as its taste. It's a simple yet tasty soup full of goodness. The ginger brings a real note of warmth to the dish and is a flavour that can be added gradually until children get used to the taste.

Ingredients:

750 g carrots

1 medium potato

1.2 l vegetable stock

Seasoning (salt, if desired, and pepper to taste)

Optional extras:

4 cm piece of fresh ginger

2 tbsp single cream

Peel and chop the carrots, potato (and ginger if you're using this ingredient, remembering to keep the pieces of ginger large enough that you can remove them later – into quarters should do it). Place the carrots, potato (and ginger) in a pan and cover with the vegetable stock. Bring to the boil and then simmer for 20 minutes. Remove from the heat and take out the ginger (if used). Transfer the ingredients into a blender and blend until a smooth consistency is achieved. Season according to taste, and stir in the cream, if desired.

Tip: Getting your child to help with the preparation of a meal is a great way of engaging them with food and eating – ask them to complete this recipe by pouring a swirl of cream into the soup.

CHICKEN SOUP

There's nothing like the hug you get from a lovely bowl of chicken soup, especially if you're feeling under the weather. If your child is disinclined to eat 'joined-up meat' this is a good recipe for providing protein without a struggle.

Ingredients:

1 large onion

1 leek

1 large potato

2 tbsp cooking oil (vegetable or olive)

450 g skinless chicken breasts

1.2 l chicken stock

Seasoning (salt, if desired, and pepper to taste)

Optional extras: 1 tbsp of both chopped parsley and thyme (fresh herbs are preferable but dried will be fine – mixed herbs will suffice if that's what's in your larder).

Peel and chop the onion, wash, trim and slice the leek, peel and chop the potato into small chunks. Heat the oil in a large saucepan on a medium heat. Add the onions and gently fry for 3 minutes until softened then add the leek and fry for a further five minutes, stirring all the while.

Trim and chop the chicken breasts into evenly sized, small chunks then add to the saucepan, stirring the pieces in with the onions and leek. Then add the potato and stock (and herbs if using), and seasoning if desired. Bring to the boil, then simmer on a lower heat for 25 minutes until the chicken is tender and cooked through.

This soup can be served as is, or, if you need to 'hide' the ingredients remove from the heat and leave to cool then blitz in a food processor until smooth, or use a hand blender before returning to the pan to reheat on a low heat for 5 minutes. For a 'cream of' version, stir in the cream at the end of cooking and continue to gently heat for a further 2 minutes.

CREAM OF TOMATO SOUP

The cheery promise of this warm and invitingly coloured soup does not fail to deliver and is always a welcome treat, especially when served with warm crusty bread.

Ingredients:

1 large onion

700 g fresh tomatoes, or 2 x 400 g tins of chopped tomatoes

2 tbsp cooking oil (vegetable or olive)

1.2 l chicken or vegetable stock

Seasoning (salt, if desired, and pepper to taste)

Optional extra: 100 ml single cream.

Peel and finely chop the onion. If you are using fresh tomatoes, first remove the skins and the stems and chop them finely too. (The best way of peeling a tomato is to cut into the fruit to break the skin, then place them in a bowl, pour boiling water over them and leave them to stand for a few minutes.

Remove the tomatoes from the water. Where you've cut into the skin it will start to peel back – you can now start removing the skins from these naturally peeled back areas with ease.)

Gently heat the oil on a low heat in a large saucepan, then add the onion and gently fry until it's softened. Add tomatoes, stock and seasoning (if desired), bring to the boil briefly then reduce the heat and simmer for 15 minutes.

Serve as is if you prefer a slightly chunkier version, or leave to cool then blitz in a food processor, or use a hand blender until smooth before returning to the pan to reheat on a low heat for 5 minutes. Stir the cream in to the soup just before serving if you would like a creamier, smoother soup (optional).

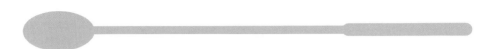

" All three of my children ate anything as babies/
toddlers then started to go off things as they
got a bit older. However, their tastes are
improving with each of them now eating some
fruit and vegetables, and the older two even
eating salad. "

CATHY, MUM OF THREE BOYS,
AGED 15, 13 AND 9

> I don't like meat because I don't like eating animals.

BEN, AGED 9

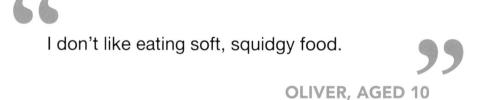

> I don't like eating soft, squidgy food.

OLIVER, AGED 10

35

CURRIED SWEET POTATO SOUP

This sweet and naturally creamy soup is easy on the palate for children. Again, this soup provides a good way of introducing new flavours and you can do this gradually by adding more heat to the dish along the way as your child grows to enjoy the spicy flavours.

Ingredients:

1 large onion

750 g sweet potatoes

2 tbsp cooking oil (vegetable or olive)

1–2 tsp curry powder

1.2 l chicken or vegetable stock

Seasoning (salt, if desired, and pepper to taste)

Peel and chop the onion and the sweet potatoes. Heat the oil in a large saucepan, then fry the onion until soft and translucent. Stir in the curry powder and cook through for a further few minutes. Add the sweet potato and stock. Bring to the boil, then reduce heat and simmer for 15 minutes until the potato is tender.

Remove the soup from the heat, season (if desired), then cool briefly before blitzing until smooth with a blender.

LEEK AND POTATO SOUP

Onions and leeks are often off-putting for children due to their texture but it can be a real advantage to get children accustomed to their flavour because onions are an integral part of many recipes. This winter warmer is a good way of introducing this flavour.

Ingredients:

1 large onion

2 leeks

2 medium potatoes

2 tbsp cooking oil (vegetable or olive)

1.2 l chicken or vegetable stock

Seasoning (salt, if desired, and pepper to taste)

Optional extra: 150 ml double cream or crème fraîche.

Peel and slice the onion, trim and slice the leeks, then peel and chop the potatoes into small chunks. Heat the oil in a large pan and gently fry the onions, potatoes and leeks for 3–4 minutes until they start to soften; stir from time to time.

Add the stock and bring to the boil then reduce heat and simmer until the vegetables are tender. Season to taste.

Leave to cool then blitz in a food processor until smooth, or use a hand blender.

Stir in the cream or crème fraîche if desired then heat through and serve.

PARSNIP AND APPLE SOUP

The sweet taste of this root vegetable is often a winner with kids, and it marries very well with apple.

Ingredients:

1 large onion

1 apple

750 g parsnips

2 tbsp cooking oil (vegetable or olive)

1.2 l chicken or vegetable stock

Seasoning (salt, if desired, and pepper to taste)

Peel and chop the onion, apple and parsnips (remember to core the apple). Heat the oil in a large saucepan, then gently fry the onion for about 5 minutes until it has softened. Then add the apple and parsnips to the pan and fry gently for a couple of minutes. Add the stock and bring to the boil, then simmer for 30 minutes. Transfer the soup into a blender and blend until smooth. Season and serve with fresh crusty bread.

TOP TIP

Don't assume they won't like food – raise your expectations and don't be afraid to try out some unusual tastes.

PEA AND HAM SOUP

As a parent you'll love that this soup has a lot going for it in terms of a balanced meal, yet it cleverly hides those little jewels – peas – that many children struggle with.

Ingredients:

1 large onion

1 large potato

2 tbsp cooking oil (vegetable or olive)

1.2 l chicken or vegetable stock

500 g frozen peas

200 g lean ham

Seasoning (salt, if desired, and pepper to taste)

Peel and finely chop the onion, peel and cube the potato. Heat the oil in a large saucepan, then fry the onion until soft and translucent. Add the potato, and cook gently for another 5 minutes. Add the stock to the pan, bring to the boil and simmer for 10 minutes or until the potatoes are soft. Add the peas, bring to the boil and wait for the peas to rise to the surface, then remove pan from heat.

Leave to cool then blitz in a food processor until smooth, or use a hand blender then tear the ham into rough pieces and stir into the pan. Bring the soup back to a simmer, then season (if desired).

TOP TIP

Be realistic when trying to introduce new flavours to your child, and remember not many adults like everything so don't expect the world.

SPICED LENTIL SOUP

This is a great soup for children who are reluctant to eat meat as lentils are a great source of protein.

Ingredients:

1 medium onion

2 celery sticks

1 medium carrot

1 garlic clove

1 tbsp cooking oil (vegetable or olive)

2 tsp garam masala curry powder

1.2 l vegetable stock

1 x 400 g can of chopped tomatoes

175 g split red lentils

2 tsp tomato purée

Seasoning (salt, if desired, and pepper)

Peel and chop the onion, celery and carrot, peel and crush the garlic. Heat the oil in a deep saucepan, then fry the onion until soft and translucent. Stir in the garlic and garam masala and cook through for a further few minutes. Add the carrots and celery and cook for another 5 minutes. Then add the stock, tomatoes, lentils and tomato purée. Bring to the boil, then reduce heat, add seasoning (if desired) and simmer for 20 minutes until the lentils are soft.

Remove the soup from the heat, leave to cool then blitz in a food processor until smooth, or use a hand blender.

VEGETABLE SOUP

This is a corker of a soup, one that will make you feel great if your child likes it as it's packed full of goodness and there are no limits as to what vegetables you can use – those listed below are just a guideline.

Ingredients:

1 medium onion

1 medium carrot

1 medium leek

2 cabbage leaves

1 medium courgette

2 tbsp cooking oil (vegetable or olive)

1.2 l vegetable stock

1 bay leaf

Seasoning (salt, if desired, and pepper to taste)

Peel and chop the onion and carrot into small chunks, wash, trim and slice the leek, roughly chop the cabbage, top and tail and slice the courgette.

Heat the oil in a large saucepan, then gently fry the onion for about 5 minutes or until it has softened. Then add the leek, cabbage, courgette and carrot and fry for a further 10 minutes. Add the stock, bay leaf and seasoning, bring to the boil, then simmer for 30 minutes. Remove the bay leaf before serving. Leave to cool then blitz in a food processor until smooth, or use a hand blender if you want to disguise the vegetable bounty within this soup. Reheat before serving.

Optional: This is one of the recipes where you can begin to make the texture less smooth once your child approves of the flavour until, finally, the soup need not be blitzed at all.

MAIN DISHES

FISHCAKES

This recipe is a great way of disguising fish from a reluctant eater. Fish can be very filling so when you combine it with potato, make sure that the cakes are a size that's manageable for your child.

Ingredients:

3 large potatoes

20 g butter (for mash)

400 g mixed filleted fish (cod, coley, salmon, pollock, hake, haddock – for a stronger flavour smoked fish can be used)

250 ml milk (for poaching fish)

4 spring onions (optional)

1 tbsp fresh dill (optional)

6 tbsp cooking oil (vegetable or olive) – 3 tbsp for binding, 3 tbsp for frying

Seasoning (salt, if desired, and pepper to taste)

2 eggs

125 g breadcrumbs

Optional: To add flavour to this dish, finely chop the spring onions and the dill and mix in with the fish and mash mixture. You can buy ready-made breadcrumbs or you can use up slightly stale bread by blitzing it in a blender for a home-made alternative.

Peel, chop and boil the potatoes, then mash with the butter and set aside to cool in a medium-sized mixing bowl.

Cut the fish into evenly sized pieces, making sure to remove any bones you find. Place the milk and fish in a shallow frying pan and gently simmer on a low heat until the fish is opaque, then remove from the hob and allow to cool.

Flake fish into the potato (along with spring onions and dill, if using). Add 3 tbsp of oil to bind ingredients together and season if desired. Once thoroughly mixed, divide ingredients into 12 equal-sized fishcakes (or to a size to suit your child).

Break the eggs into a bowl and lightly beat until they are thoroughly mixed. Place the breadcrumbs in a separate bowl. Then, take each individual fishcake and dip it into the egg, then roll in breadcrumbs until each is fully coated in crumbs, then place each fishcake on a plate.

Heat oil in a frying pan on a medium heat and add fishcakes. Fry each for 10 minutes, turning regularly until each side is browned then remove from heat, drain on kitchen roll and serve with your choice of vegetables.

TOP TIP

Offer a new food only when your child is hungry and rested. There's no point trying to 'persuade' a child to try something they're unsure about if they are tired and fractious.

FISH PIE

For fish-loving families this one's a winner. Keep it simple or spruce it up a little – whichever way it's hearty, healthy and utterly delicious.

Ingredients:

750 g potatoes

600 g filleted haddock, whiting, cod or a mixture of any of them

1 medium onion

300 ml whole milk

6 peppercorns

1 bay leaf (both the bay leaf and peppercorns add great flavour to the cooking milk but won't make it into the final pie!)

Seasoning to taste (salt, if desired, and pepper)

25 g butter

25 g plain flour

2 tbsp cream

Optional: For a little more luxury (and protein) in your pie, add quartered hard-boiled eggs before cooking, and 1 tbsp of chopped parsley.

Preheat the oven to 180°C/350°F/gas mark 4.

Peel and chop potatoes, place in a pan and cover with water, bring to the boil then simmer for 20 minutes before straining and mashing with a little butter. Set aside to cool.

Lay the fish fillets in a roasting pan.

Peel and chop the onion, then place in a pan and heat with the milk, peppercorns, bay leaf and seasoning if desired for about 5 minutes (or you can warm these ingredients in a jug in the microwave for about 2 minutes).

Pour the mixture over the fish and cook in the oven for about 10 to 15 minutes, until the fish is firm.

Strain off the milk, reserving it for the sauce. Flake the fish into a 2 litre ovenproof dish, add the eggs and sprinkle over the parsley if using.

Heat the butter in a saucepan, stir in the flour and cook for 1 minute. Draw off the heat and gradually add the reserved milk, mixing the sauce continually to avoid lumps forming.

Return to the heat and stir, bringing slowly to the boil. Taste and season as desired. Stir in the cream and pour over the fish, gently mixing it with a palette knife or spoon.

Spread a layer of mashed potatoes on the top and mark with a fork in a criss-cross pattern. Dot with butter.

Place the ovenproof dish in the oven and cook for about 20 minutes, or until the top is golden brown.

" My child tried a lot of things that he would ordinarily decline at home through eating school dinners. "

HILARY, MUM OF 8-YEAR-OLD BOY

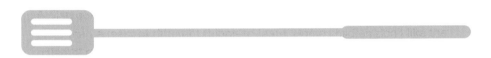

" I always insist that Kyle tries a little bit of whatever we're eating before he can say he doesn't like it. "

AMY, MUM OF KYLE, AGED 7

" I don't believe fussy eating is to do with the parents and how they feed their children. Kai, my eldest son, eats pretty much anything, whereas my youngest, Cayden, is very fussy and hardly eats anything, only plain foods and definitely nothing with a sauce. "

DAVE, DAD OF TWO BOYS,
AGED 10 AND 5

TUNA, POTATO AND EGG SALAD

This is the perfect protein-packed meal that can be ready in minutes. You can add extras or keep it simple.

Ingredients:

400 g new potatoes, halved

4 large eggs, quartered

1 romaine lettuce, leaves separated and washed

2 x 160 g tins of tuna

2 tbsp reduced fat mayonnaise

Optional: To make a proper tuna Niçoise, add any, some or all of the following ingredients to your salad: cooked green beans, cherry tomatoes halved, a handful of black olives and drained and rinsed anchovy fillets.

Bring a pan of water to the boil. Add the potatoes and the eggs, and cook the eggs for 7–10 minutes (depending on how hard boiled you like your eggs) and the potatoes for 10–12 minutes. When cooked for your desired amount of time, scoop the eggs out of the pan and run under cold water until cool. Drain the potatoes and also leave to cool.

Cut the potatoes in half and peel the eggs and cut into quarters. Arrange the lettuce leaves on plates or in shallow bowls. Scatter over the potatoes and egg quarters.

Flake the tuna into chunks and scatter over the salad. Mix the mayonnaise and 1 tbsp cold water in a bowl until smooth. Drizzle over the salad and serve.

HOME-MADE FISH FINGERS

This dish is one that allows you to use the fish of your choice and is a great one for getting your children to help with the preparation.

Ingredients:

300 g skinless filleted white fish (haddock, whiting, cod, pollock, etc.)

1 large egg, beaten

50 g breadcrumbs

½ tbsp cooking oil (vegetable or olive)

Preheat the oven to 200°C/390°F/ gas mark 6.

Cut the fish into equal-sized portions (fingers).

Break the egg into a bowl and lightly beat until thoroughly mixed. Place the breadcrumbs in a separate bowl. Then, take each individual portion of fish and dip it into the egg until fully coated, then coat in breadcrumbs and place on a plate to stand.

Grease a baking tray using the oil and place the fish on the tray and cook in the oven for 15 minutes, turning the fish halfway through. Remove from the oven and serve immediately.

TOP TIP

Try not to force the issue;
if you insist that a child eats
something you are bound to
confront their iron will. Instead,
try alternative approaches,
for instance using distraction
as a technique to
make it fun.

SALMON BURGERS

Fish can be off-putting to children due to its smell and the texture. Changing the appearance of the fish into a well-loved burger form is a good way of introducing this low fat source of protein into your child's diet.

Ingredients:

450 g raw salmon fillet

1 small onion

6 tbsp cooking oil (vegetable or olive) – 3 tbsp for binding, 3 tbsp for frying

Seasoning to taste (salt, if desired, and pepper)

2 tbsp plain flour

Optional: If you'd like to spice up your burgers, add 1 tbsp of finely chopped dill, capers or gherkins to the mix.

Remove all skin and bones from the salmon, chop the fish into pieces and blitz in a food processor to create a rough texture, not a purée.

Peel and finely dice the onion. If your child doesn't like 'onion bits' you can purée the onion instead or substitute the onion with frozen puréed cubes (see page 21 for instructions). Heat the oil in a large frying pan, add onions and gently fry until they become translucent. Remove from the heat and transfer into a mixing bowl and allow to cool. Add salmon and seasoning to the onions and combine ingredients until well mixed (you can do this by hand if you prefer). If you are using puréed onions cut out the first frying stage and simply bind the fish and onions together with the oil. If you are spicing up your burger, mix in the added ingredients at this stage.

With floured hands, divide ingredients into four equal portions, and shape each into a ball. Roll each ball in the remaining flour and flatten each ball into a burger shape.

Heat the further measure of oil in a frying pan on a medium heat and place each burger in the frying pan and gently fry for approximately 15–20 minutes, turning regularly to avoid burning.

Serve in a bun, or simply as it stands.

TOP TIP

It's quite normal for children to want to be able to identify the food they are eating, and although loads of good stuff can be masked in a sauce, some children can find sauces off-putting.

CHEESY PASTA WITH SWEETCORN

Quick to prepare and packed with flavour, this dish makes a satisfying meal in minutes.

Ingredients:

300 g pasta

100 g sweetcorn (frozen or tinned)

100 g Cheddar cheese

20 g butter

1 tbsp plain flour

250 ml semi-skimmed milk

Seasoning (salt, if desired, and pepper to taste)

Preheat the oven to 200°C/390°F/ gas mark 6.

Place the pasta in a large saucepan and cover with water. Bring to the boil, then simmer for 10 minutes. Add the sweetcorn and continue cooking for a further 5 minutes. Drain and set aside. While the pasta is cooking, make a cheese sauce. Firstly grate the Cheddar and set aside. Melt the butter in a small saucepan, but don't let it brown. Then stir in the flour and cook gently for a couple of minutes, trying to avoid getting any lumps. Remove from the heat and mix in a little of the milk to form a paste. Continue to stir in small amounts of milk at a time until the white sauce has a smooth consistency – the milk has to be added gradually otherwise the sauce will end up being lumpy. When all the milk has been added, return the pan to the heat to thicken, stirring to avoid it sticking to the pan. Now add the grated cheese to the white sauce when you return it to the heat and stir. Simmer for 5 minutes or so, then season.

Mix the pasta and sweetcorn into the cheese sauce then place into an ovenproof dish and cook in the oven for 10 minutes before serving.

TOP TIP

A dish containing just a few elements can seem more manageable and appealing for a child than a feast of things to taste – try to keep things simple.

MACARONI CHEESE

Macaroni cheese is a classic dish that can be bought in tins, pre-prepared or frozen but nothing compares to making it yourself and, in doing so, with trial and error, you can temper the recipe to the strength of cheese flavour your child will like best.

Ingredients:

300 g dried macaroni

40 g butter

40 g plain flour

600 ml milk

300 g grated Cheddar

Cook the macaroni in a pan of boiling water for 8–10 minutes; drain well and set aside.

Melt the butter in a large saucepan. Add the flour and stir constantly to form a roux, and continue to cook for a few minutes. Gradually stir in the milk, a little at a time to avoid lumpiness. Cook for 10–15 minutes to a thickened and smooth sauce then remove the pan from the heat and add about two thirds of the cheese, and stir in until melted.

Add the macaroni to the sauce and mix well to make sure the pasta is thoroughly coated. Transfer to a deep ovenproof dish.

Preheat the grill to hot, sprinkle over the remaining cheese and place the dish under the grill. Cook until the cheese is browned and bubbling. Serve immediately.

CHORIZO PASTA

This may sound a bit far-fetched for a child with simple tastes but there's something about the smoky saltiness of this dish that seems to appeal to those who often struggle with spicy flavours.

Ingredients:

200 g boneless and skinless chicken breast

200 g chorizo sausage

350 g broccoli

350 g pasta (penne or fusilli works best)

2 tbsp cooking oil (vegetable or olive)

Seasoning (salt, if desired, and pepper to taste)

90 g pesto

Firstly prepare the meat: chop the chicken into even bite-sized chunks then skin the chorizo sausage if necessary, and chop into small pieces. Chop the broccoli, broken into equal sized florets.

Bring a large pan of water to the boil then add the pasta shapes and bring back to boil, reduce heat and simmer for 10–12 minutes. Add the broccoli to the boiling water after 9 minutes. Drain when both the pasta and broccoli are al dente, then return to the pan and cover with a lid.

In the meantime, heat the oil in a large frying pan and add the chorizo sausage pieces. Fry the sausage for 3–4 minutes on a fairly high heat to release juices. Remove sausages from frying pan and set aside.

Add the chicken pieces to the frying pan containing the chorizo juices and fry at a fairly high heat for 7–10 minutes until cooked through. Season, if required. Stir frequently to avoid chicken browning on one side only, then remove from heat.

Now place the pasta, broccoli, chorizo and chicken in a larger frying pan or wok and stir the pesto into the ingredients so they have a good covering. Gently reheat until hot.

TOP TIP

It's quite normal for children to be 'scared' of some foods – try to be sensitive to this when you introduce something new or unusual. Assume that eating habits will change slowly as it takes time to break down the barriers that have been formed against eating certain foodstuffs.

LASAGNE

This dish takes a little time, but the difference between this and many shop-bought versions is huge in terms of the texture and flavour it packs. We promise many previously reluctant lasagne eaters will be converted to this Italian classic.

Ingredients:

1 large onion

2 cloves of garlic

2 tbsp cooking oil (vegetable or olive)

500 g minced beef

1 x 400 g can of chopped tomatoes

2 tsp oregano

125 ml beef stock

2 tbsp tomato purée

Seasoning to taste (salt, if desired, and pepper)

1 packet of lasagne ('no pre-cooking required' type)

Preheat oven to 200°C/390°F/gas mark 6

Peel and chop the onion and garlic. Heat the oil in a saucepan and fry the onion and garlic for 5 minutes, then add the mince and cook thoroughly, stirring from time to time to avoid clumps forming. Next, add the tomatoes, oregano, beef stock, tomato purée and seasoning and bring to the boil, then simmer for 15–20 minutes.

If your child does not like 'bits', onion ice cubes can be used in place of raw onion (see page 21). If you know that your child will pick out every single onion or tomato lump from this meal then opt for a blitzed version instead. Defrost the onion ice cube, heat 1 tsp oil in a large frying pan then gently fry the onion until soft and then add the garlic and fry for a further 3 minutes until translucent. Add the chopped tomatoes and seasoning, bring to the boil, reduce heat and allow to simmer for 10 minutes. Blitz the sauce with a hand blender. Then, gently fry the mince off in a frying pan until browned and mix in the tomato mixture with the beef stock and tomato purée. Simmer to reduce as above.

While the meat sauce is reducing, prepare the cheese sauce (see cheese sauce recipe on page 26.

Grease a shallow baking dish then add a layer of meat sauce followed by a layer of lasagne, followed by a layer of cheese sauce. Continue this formation until you have used up your mixtures, making sure you finish with the cheese sauce. Sprinkle grated cheese on top.

Bake for 30–40 minutes, until the top is lightly browned.

> With vegetables that I know he will eat I tell him he must finish them if he's to have a dessert.

CAROLINE, MUM OF GEORGE, AGED 7

> I made all of their baby food, and both boys would eat fruit and veg in a purée. I then struggled to get them to eat joined-up raw or cooked fruit and veg.

CHRIS, DAD OF SAM AND JACK,
AGED 6 AND 9

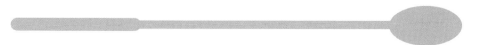

"
I was brought up to eat what was put in front of me. If I didn't, I'd go hungry. There were no snacks in the house except fruit. I'm not as strict on my kids but I do feel that I have not done them any favours by being soft.
"

MANDY, MUM OF GEMMA AND HOPE,
AGED 7 AND 5

TOP TIP

Telling your child to 'eat it, it's good for you' rarely reaps a positive response. Try using alternative techniques to describe the food, for example 'try this it's really sweet/ juicy', etc.

BUTTERY GARLIC PASTA

This dish really doesn't get much simpler, but it's hard to get much tastier!

Ingredients:

2 tbsp Parmesan cheese

1 clove of garlic

25 g butter

2 tbsp olive oil

350 g of spaghetti or your favourite pasta

Optional extras: 1 handful of chopped basil or parsley.

Grate the Parmesan cheese.

To make the spaghetti sauce, first peel and crush the garlic, and fry gently in butter and olive oil over a medium-low heat just until the garlic is soft but not browned.

Chop the basil or parsley, if desired, and stir in with the garlic then cook for 2 minutes (stirring constantly) until the herbs are limp but still green.

Pour the sauce hot over cooked pasta, any variety to suit your tastes, toss lightly to coat and top with the Parmesan cheese before serving.

CREAMY SAUSAGE PASTA

This yummy dish truly delivers on flavour and creaminess and is simple to prepare. Good quality sausages are a must.

Ingredients:

1 clove of garlic

1 medium onion

1 tbsp cooking oil (vegetable or olive)

4 thick pork sausages

1 x 400 g can of chopped tomatoes

50 g Parmesan

2 tbsp cream or mascarpone

350 g tagliatelle or your favourite pasta

Seasoning to taste (salt, if desired, and pepper)

Optional: The more adventurous will find a handful of herbs, particularly finely chopped fresh rosemary, really enhances the taste.

Peel and crush the garlic and peel and finely chop the onion. Heat the oil in a pan then add the onion and gently fry for 3 minutes. Add the garlic and fry for another minute or so.

Next remove the sausage meat from the skin and crumble the meat into the pan with the onions and garlic, and cook together for a further 6–7 minutes to ensure the sausage meat is lightly browned.

Add the can of chopped tomatoes (and any herbs if you're using them), stir together well, then let the mixture simmer gently for a further 15 minutes.

Lastly, add the majority of the Parmesan (leaving a handful aside for the topping) and the cream or mascarpone to the mix, stir together well. Serve with the pasta, either mix it together, served on top or to the side – the choice is yours! Sprinkle the remaining Parmesan over the dish and you're done.

SPAGHETTI BOLOGNESE

From its start point as the most simple of dishes it can be embellished as a child's tastes develop. You'll most likely settle on your own favourite version, tailored to meet your tastes.

Ingredients:

2 cloves of garlic

1 medium onion

1 medium carrot

1 stick of celery

50 g streaky or smoked bacon

1 tbsp cooking oil (vegetable or olive)

350 g minced beef (lean is best)

1 x 400 g can of chopped tomatoes

2 tsp dried oregano

A generous splash of red wine if you have some

2 tbsp tomato purée

350 g of spaghetti or your favourite pasta

Seasoning to taste (salt, if desired, and pepper)

(Serve sauce with spaghetti or other pasta shapes if preferred – use approximately 80 g dried pasta per person.)

Peel and crush the garlic and peel and finely chop the onion, carrot and celery. Dice the bacon.

Heat the oil in a large frying pan then add the onions and gently fry for 3 minutes, then add the garlic, carrot, celery and bacon and fry for a further 3–4 minutes (if you've tried but your child really will not eat identifiable vegetable lumps, blitz the mixture at this stage). Add the minced beef and cook on a high heat for a further 3 minutes until all the meat is browned. Stir in the tomatoes, oregano and wine (if you are using) and bring to the boil then reduce the heat, stir in tomato purée and season to taste. Leave to simmer for about 45 minutes. If 'green bits' are a deal-breaker with your children, omit the oregano.

Remember to prepare your pasta so that it's ready to serve at the same time as the sauce is ready.

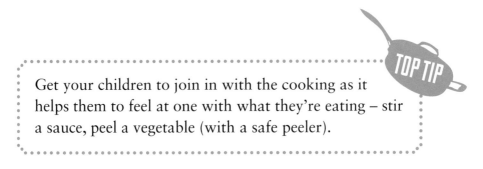

Get your children to join in with the cooking as it helps them to feel at one with what they're eating – stir a sauce, peel a vegetable (with a safe peeler).

TUNA PASTA BAKE

This quick and easy dish is a great meal to prepare when you're short of time and you're relying on the contents of your larder.

Ingredients:

350 g broccoli

350 g pasta (penne or fusilli works best)

2 x 160 g tins of tuna

1 x 400 g can of chopped tomatoes

Seasoning to taste (salt, if desired, and pepper)

100 g Cheddar cheese

Preheat oven to 180°C/350°F/ gas mark 4.

Chop the broccoli, broken into equal sized florets.

Bring a large pan of water to the boil then add the pasta and bring back to the boil, reduce heat and simmer for 10–12 minutes, adding the broccoli to the water after about 5 minutes. Drain when the pasta and broccoli are al dente. Drain any oil or brine from the tuna then mix into the pasta and broccoli along with the chopped tomatoes. Season to taste.

Place the mixture into an ovenproof dish and cook in a preheated oven for 10 minutes. Grate the cheese and sprinkle over the pasta mix and cook for a further 10 minutes before serving.

CHINESE BARBECUE CHICKEN

This dish is best started a couple of hours ahead of serving as the meat benefits from being marinated. For optimum taste leave overnight if you can. Although this is a great dish for the BBQ it can be cooked in the oven.

Ingredients:

3 cm piece of fresh ginger

1 clove of garlic

2 tbsp clear honey

2 tsp Chinese five spice

2 tsp soy sauce

1 tbsp sesame oil

4 chicken drumsticks

4 chicken wings

Preheat oven to 180°C/350°F/gas mark 4 (unless you are barbecuing).

Peel and grate the ginger, peel and crush the garlic then mix with the honey, spices, soy and oil. Place the chicken in an ovenproof dish, coat with the honey mixture and leave to marinate for at least half an hour in the fridge. The sooner this is done the better if you want a really rich taste (left overnight in the fridge for absolute best results).

If you are using an oven, place the ovenproof dish into the preheated oven and cook for about 30 minutes, turning occasionally and basting with the marinade and juices until thoroughly sticky and golden. Check the chicken is cooked through.

If you are barbecuing the dish, place the chicken on the barbecue over medium-hot coals and cook for about 20 minutes, making sure you cook the chicken all the way through. To check, pierce a drumstick with a skewer: if the juices are still pink, carry on cooking.

CRISPY BATTERED CHICKEN GOUJONS

There's a pretty good chance that this fast food favourite will be a hit with the younger ones, but make it with this straightforward, yet tasty recipe, and it could just be a winner with the whole family.

Ingredients:

Sunflower oil, for deep-frying

450 g skinless chicken breasts

300 ml milk

4 tbsp plain flour

Seasoning (salt, if desired, and pepper to taste)

Heat a deep fat fryer (if you have one) filled with sunflower oil to 170°C. Alternatively, pour the oil into a large saucepan to a depth of 2 cm and heat on a high setting on the hob – to see if the oil is hot enough add a chunk of bread to the oil and if it cooks and browns then the oil is ready.

Cut the chicken into strips. Pour the milk into a small bowl. Mix the flour in another bowl and season.

Working in batches to ensure they don't stick together, dip the chicken pieces in the milk and then in the flour to coat. Shake off any excess flour and deep-fry for 4–5 minutes or until crisp, golden and cooked through. Drain well on kitchen paper. This dish is delicious served with a fresh green salad, or raw vegetables chopped into batons (red and yellow pepper, carrots and cucumber work well).

TOP TIP

Some children don't like
the different elements of the dish
they're eating to be touching each other.
If this is the case, simply arrange food in a
way that means your child is happy to eat it.

The way food is presented can be a deal-
breaker. For instance, too much on a plate
can be a complete turn-off for a child
as it can seem like a daunting task
for a small appetite to tackle.

CHICKEN CASSEROLE

This one-pot wonder, served with mashed potato, pasta, rice or couscous provides a great balanced meal that all the family can enjoy.

Ingredients:

1 onion

2 large carrots

750 ml chicken stock

8 small boneless chicken thighs

1 tbsp cooking oil (vegetable or olive)

2 tbsp plain flour

Seasoning (salt, if desired, and pepper to taste)

Optional: Switch onion for leek for a more delicate flavour.

Peel and finely chop the onion and carrots. Heat the stock. Remove the skin from the chicken and discard it.

Heat the oil in a casserole or wide pan with a lid, add the chicken thighs and fry until browned. Stir in the onion with the flour and gradually stir in the stock, making sure no lumps form. Add the carrots, bring to the boil and then cover with the lid and simmer for 30 minutes. Remove the lid and simmer for a further 15 minutes. Season to taste.

If you need to 'hide' the onions and carrots, simply remove the chicken from the dish and set aside under some foil to keep hot, blitz the remaining ingredients until smooth, then replace the chicken into the casserole dish/wide pan.

CHICKEN KIEV

This buttery classic dish makes a great occasional treat with its wonderful texture and flavour sensation.

Ingredients:

2 cloves of garlic

175 g butter

2 tbsp lemon juice

Seasoning (salt, if desired, and pepper to taste)

1 egg

10–12 tbsp breadcrumbs

2 tbsp plain flour

4 large chicken breasts

2 tbsp cooking oil (vegetable or olive)

Optional: Add a handful of chopped parsley to your butter mix.

Preheat the oven to 200°C/390°F/ gas mark 6.

Peel and finely chop the garlic then soften the butter slightly in a bowl and mix in the garlic, lemon juice and seasoning.

Take three small bowls – lightly beat the egg in one, place the breadcrumbs in the second, and the flour in a third.

Make a pocket in the chicken breast by cutting lengthways with a sharp knife, leaving a couple of centimetres at either end of the breast. Push the butter mixture into the pocket in each chicken breast.

Roll the chicken breasts in flour then dip them into the egg, then into the bowl containing breadcrumbs until each breast is coated completely.

Shake off any excess.

Heat the oil in a frying pan and fry the chicken breasts on all sides until lightly browned. Transfer the chicken to an ovenproof dish and bake in the oven for 18–20 minutes, or until golden brown and completely cooked through.

TOP TIP

Learn to judge the difference between your child's fussiness versus their having a genuine dislike for a particular foodstuff.

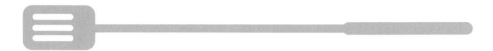

" My daughter had more explorative tastes as she got older, trying things like olives and a range of seafood, mussels, octopus and squid – going on holiday to a foreign country and eating out in restaurants helped this. "

MARIA, MUM OF ELLA, AGED 9

"Fussy eating is exaggerated by the parents' fear that a child is not eating enough. I've found that giving a child countless choices of food rather than a small and manageable selection at mealtimes, or restricting the amount of time they have to finish their meal will, if you persevere, reap better results than trying to appease a child's eating desires. "

EMMA, MUM OF TWO AND
A REGISTERED CHILDMINDER

CHICKEN KORMA

This is a bit of a cheat really as it does rely on a pre-bought jar, but it is one of the quickest and easiest meals to knock together when you're in a rush. The mild nature of this curry opens the door for an enormous range of other spicy meals (not to mention trips to Indian restaurants or treat takeaways when you fancy a night off from cooking).

Ingredients:

1 large onion

450 g skinless chicken breasts

Cooking oil (vegetable or olive)

90 g korma paste

1 x 400 g can of coconut milk

Seasoning (salt, if desired, pepper to taste)

Peel and finely chop the onion. Cut the chicken breasts into bite-sized cubes.

Heat the oil in a large frying pan or heavy bottomed saucepan, add the onion and fry until soft. Add the chicken and fry for 3–4 minutes until they've changed colour. Add the korma paste and fry for a further 1–2 minutes. If you are using ice cube puréed onion in place of fresh onion, defrost the requisite number of cubes (see page 21 for advice on this) and add to the chicken with the korma paste. Mix in the coconut milk, season and bring to the boil, then simmer gently for 20 minutes.

Serve with boiled rice and peas.

TOP TIP

Involving your child in
the decision making about menus
can help to make them more interested
in the food they eat. Ask them to choose
whether they'd prefer peas or carrots with
the dish, pasta or potatoes.

Sometimes, however, offering a choice of what,
or how much, to eat can be the road to disaster
when a child is fussy – you'll have to get the
measure of your child to know whether or
not to offer a choice, or simply present a
dish as a fait accompli so that you
don't have to have a battle
of negotiation.

CHICKEN WITH MOZZARELLA AND PARMA HAM
(chizella, as it's known to us)

This is an unlikely sounding combination for those with a limited palate but it has proved to be a winner and has become a firm family favourite.

Ingredients:

1 large ball of mozzarella

4 small chicken breasts

Seasoning (salt, if desired, pepper to taste)

Pesto (1–2 tsp per breast)

Basil leaves (optional)

Parma ham (3–4 slices per chicken breast)

Cooking oil (vegetable or olive)

Preheat oven to 200°C/390°F/ gas mark 6.

Slice the mozzarella into 2 cm wide batons.

Cover chicken breasts with cling film leaving a generous amount each side of the breast then use a rolling pin to gently hammer the chicken to flatten it out to a thickness of approximately 4 mm – this process helps tenderise the meat.

Open the cling film to expose chicken breast, season if desired. Smother breast with pesto and place the mozzarella pieces in the centre of the chicken, leaving 2 cm at each end of the breast. (If using basil leaves, place on top of the mozzarella – they do add flavour and texture but if your child fears green 'bits' these could be a stretch too far.)

Take one long edge of each chicken breast and fold over the mozzarella/pesto mix then roll into a sausage shape. Squish the ends of the breast in to create a seal. The cling film can be used to help create a tight sausage.

Take the Parma ham and lay out on a chopping board so that each strip overlaps the other, then place the chicken sausage (having removed the cling film) in the centre of the strips, horizontal to their perpendicular.

Wrap the strips of ham around the chicken sausage as tightly as possible and try to fold the end in to keep the ingredients of the sausage in place.

Glaze a baking tray with olive oil and place each chicken roll on the tray and put in your preheated oven towards the top. Bake for 20–30 minutes until the ham is crisp. Remove from the oven, set aside to rest for 10 minutes and then slice each into rounds.

This dish goes very well with crunchy green beans and boiled potatoes, or a simple green salad.

TOP TIP

Make food colourful – children are often attracted by the most brightly coloured foods so try to delight them with a palette of hues.

CHICKEN PIE

This is a great dish to prepare when you're trying to use up leftovers. It can be prepared with cooked chicken, or leftover cooked turkey after Christmas.

Ingredients:

175 g cooked ham

500 g cooked chicken

1 egg

300 ml milk

25 g butter

25 g flour

Seasoning (salt, if desired, and pepper)

225 g puff pastry

Optional: Mushrooms can have an unpalatable texture for some children, if they can stomach them, they are an ideal pairing with this pie. But if you choose to use them you'll need 110 g mushrooms and an extra 25 g butter.

Preheat the oven to 190°C/375°F/ gas mark 5.

Chop the cooked ham and cooked chicken into small chunks. Break the egg and beat it lightly with 1 tbsp of the milk.

(If you are opting for mushrooms, clean and slice them, then melt your extra 25 g of butter in a saucepan, add the mushrooms and fry for 3 minutes. Transfer to a plate ready to add to the meat mixture later.)

Melt the butter in the pan. Stir in the flour to form a smooth paste. Stirring constantly, slowly add the milk and bring to the boil. Add the remaining ingredients (including the mushrooms if you desire). Cook for 3–5 minutes. Transfer to a deep, medium-sized pie dish.

Roll out the pastry until it is about 5 mm thick. Cover the pie dish with the pastry, trim off the excess and brush the top with the egg mixture. Bake in the oven for 30–35 minutes or until the pastry is deep golden brown.

CHICKEN RISOTTO

This is not one of those dishes to be left to its own devices when cooking – it takes plenty of watching and stirring but it's well worth it in the end.

Ingredients:

75 g skinless chicken breast

25 g butter

1 medium onion

1 clove of garlic

200 g rice (Arborio works best but easy cook long grain will suffice)

500 ml chicken stock

Seasoning (salt, if desired, and pepper)

Optional: This dish can be enhanced with all sorts of added extras, from peas to sweetcorn or mushrooms. If you choose to embellish the dish you'll need about 50 g of the added ingredient.

Cut the chicken into pieces. Heat the butter in a large saucepan and fry the chicken pieces for 5 minutes, then remove from the pan and put them in a bowl.

Peel and chop the onion and garlic and fry for 3–4 minutes. Add the rice to the onions and fry gently for a further minute or two.

Either use your hot home-made stock or prepare the stock using a cube and boiling water. Add the stock to the rice a little at a time, stirring all the while. Let the rice simmer gently until the stock is all absorbed and the rice is cooked. This should take about 20 minutes. Season as desired.

When the rice is cooked, add the chicken (and any other extra ingredients of your choice) and cook for a minute or so, to heat them through.

RED THAI CURRY

This mildly spicy dish offers a more fragrant taste than an Indian curry.

Ingredients:

1 tbsp cooking oil (groundnut is best for an authentic flavour but vegetable oil can be used too)

2 tbsp red Thai curry paste

4 chicken breasts

1 x 400 ml tin of coconut milk

1 cup of water

1 red pepper

2 tsp brown sugar

2 tsp grated lime rind

1 tbsp fish sauce

Optional extra: Fresh coriander.

Heat the oil in a wok or large frying pan. Add the curry paste and cook for a minute, stirring as it cooks to avoid the paste sticking to the pan.

Cut the chicken into chunks and stir-fry for 3–4 minutes until they are golden in colour, after which add the coconut milk and water. Bring to the boil, then chop and deseed the red pepper and add to the wok, then simmer for 10 minutes.

Finally, add the sugar, lime and fish sauce and cook gently for a further 5 minutes. Add chopped or torn coriander leaves to serve if you desire.

Serve with rice.

TOMATO CHICKEN

The rich colour of this sauce is very appetising for children and its Mediterranean-style flavour is enough to warm you on even the coldest winter evening.

Ingredients:

1 large onion

2 cloves of garlic

2 red peppers

4 chicken breasts

1 tbsp cooking oil (vegetable or olive)

2 x 400 g cans of chopped tomatoes

1 tbsp tomato purée

1 bay leaf

Seasoning (salt, if desired, and pepper)

Optional extras: 3 tsp oregano, 3 tsp paprika (smoked or hot smoked to spice up), 100 ml red wine.

Preheat oven:180°C/350°F/gas mark 4 if using the oven method.

Peel and finely chop the onion and garlic; core, deseed and chop the peppers into strips; cut chicken breasts into strips. Heat the oil in a large frying pan and fry the onions, pepper and garlic until softened and then add the chicken strips and fry until they begin to colour (3–4 minutes).

Add tinned tomatoes and purée, bay leaf and seasoning (and the oregano, paprika and red wine if desired).

Bring to the boil and gently simmer on the hob for 40 minutes, uncovered, adding a little water from time to time to keep the consistency liquid. Alternatively, transfer ingredients to an ovenproof dish and cook in the preheated oven for an hour (no extra water required).

Remove the bay leaf and serve with boiled rice, pasta or mashed potato.

CREAMY CHICKEN (OR TURKEY) WITH BACON

Another great way to use up leftovers from the roast, this dish can be adapted according to taste.

Ingredients:

1 medium onion

1 clove of garlic

Leftover cooked turkey or chicken

1 tbsp cooking oil (vegetable or olive)

2–3 thick rashers streaky bacon or pancetta

100–200 g frozen peas (optional)

2–3 tbsp double cream or crème fraîche

Seasoning (salt, if desired, and pepper to taste)

50 g Parmesan cheese

Peel and finely chop the onion and garlic. Chop the meat into small chunks.

Heat the oil in a frying pan and add the bacon or pancetta, and fry until just crispy. Turn the heat down, then add the onions and garlic and sweat until soft but not coloured.

Add the peas and a splash of water and allow to bubble for a couple of minutes. When the pan is almost dry again add the turkey or chicken and heat through.

Add the cream or crème fraîche and season if desired. Allow to bubble until the cream has reduced a little and the sauce has a nice coating consistency. Serve tossed with your chosen pasta, with plenty of freshly grated Parmesan.

TURKEY BURGERS

For some children the idea of fast food, especially a burger in a bun, is more appealing than the boring old stuff that's served up at home. This recipe brings fast food home, and offers a more healthy option to boot.

Ingredients:

1 small onion

6 tbsp cooking oil (vegetable or olive) – 3 tbsp for binding, 3 tbsp for frying

450 g minced turkey

Seasoning to taste (salt, if desired, and pepper)

Optional: If you'd like to spice your burgers up, optional extras can be 1 tsp smoked paprika or 1 tbsp finely chopped parsley, gherkins or capers – experiment depending on your taste.

Peel and finely dice the onion (purée, or substitute with ice cube onion purée if your child does not like 'bits' in their food).

Heat the oil in a large frying pan, add onions and gently fry until golden then transfer the contents of the frying pan into a mixing bowl. Allow to cool and add turkey mince and seasoning.

Combine ingredients until well mixed. If you are using puréed onions or ice cube puréed onions cut out the first frying stage and simply bind the meat and onions together with the oil, remembering to defrost the ice cubes ahead of use.

Divide ingredients into four equal portions, and shape each into a ball. Flatten each ball into a burger shape. Heat the further measure of oil in a frying pan on a medium heat and place each burger in the frying pan.

Cook for approximately 15–20 minutes, turning regularly to avoid burning, until juices from the burgers run clear. Drain the oil or dab the burgers on kitchen roll to remove any surplus oil. Serve in a bun, or simply as it stands with a salad.

TURKEY WITH CREAM (AND TARRAGON)

We know what you'll be thinking... tarragon, I don't think so. Believe us, this enhances the flavour of the dish perfectly, and it can be removed just before serving so your fussy eater won't even know about it!

Ingredients:

1 large onion

2 tbsp cooking oil (vegetable or olive)

400 g turkey

250 ml chicken stock

Several sprigs of fresh tarragon

Seasoning (salt, if desired, and pepper)

300 ml double cream

Peel and finely chop the onion. Heat the oil in a large frying pan and gently fry the onion until soft. Use puréed onion or ice cube onion purée if you want to avoid 'bits'. Cut the turkey into evenly sized strips and fry with the onion until it begins to take colour. Add the chicken stock, tarragon sprigs and seasoning and bring to the boil before reducing the heat and simmering for 10–15 minutes.

Once the turkey is fully cooked remove the tarragon sprigs, add the cream to the dish and cook through for a further 3 minutes until the sauce thickens. Serve with rice or pasta.

TOP TIP

If you are presenting new foods, only put one new food forward at a time. It helps if you pair a new food with a favourite food to increase your child's acceptance.

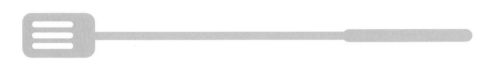

" Appearance of food doesn't have a huge effect on my child liking something, but it does have a big effect on her disliking something. "

ELLEN, MUM OF MAISIE, AGED 7

" I include things on her plate that she doesn't usually eat alongside things she does to encourage her to try new things. "

JULIAN, DAD OF HANNAH, AGED 6

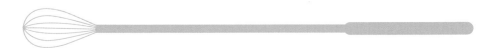

"
I've never forced our children to eat something; instead I just keep on getting them to try things because I know their tastes could change with time.
"

MURIEL, MUM OF MATHIEU, VINCENT AND ALICE

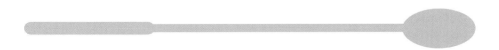

BEEF BURGERS

Another great way to bring fast food home, there's really nothing like a juicy home-made burger. Have some fun along the way and make them together.

Ingredients:

1 small onion

1 clove of garlic

1 tbsp cooking oil (vegetable or olive)

500 g lean minced beef

50 g breadcrumbs

1 egg

Seasoning (salt, if desired, and pepper)

Optional: To add flavour to the burgers any of the following ingredients can be added: 1 tsp French mustard; a dash of Tabasco sauce; a dash of Worcestershire sauce.

Peel and finely chop the onion and garlic. Heat the oil in a frying pan and gently fry the onion and garlic for 3 minutes. Leave to cool slightly. Then place all the ingredients in a bowl and mix together well (use defrosted onion ice cubes if you're worried about 'bits'). Divide the mixture into portions that suit your children, then shape each portion into something that resembles a burger. Cook under a medium grill for about 4–5 minutes on each side, depending on the thickness of the burger.

BEEF CASSEROLE

Classic comfort food, simple to prepare and almost impossible to overcook, as casseroles almost always benefit from a slower cook.

Ingredients:

1 large onion

1 clove of garlic

3 medium carrots

500 g stewing steak

40 g plain flour

Seasoning (salt, if desired, and pepper)

2 tbsp cooking oil (vegetable or olive)

500 ml beef stock

1 bay leaf

Preheat oven to 180°C/350°F/ gas mark 4.

Peel and chop the onion, garlic and carrots. Cut the meat into small bite-sized pieces and roll them in some of the flour with a little seasoning. Use a flameproof casserole dish to heat the oil on the hob, add the meat once the oil is hot then brown the meat on all sides. Remove the meat and set aside. Fry the garlic for a couple of minutes in the casserole dish. Add the rest of the flour to the pan and fry gently. Add the stock and boil until it thickens. Add the carrots and meat to the dish, with the bay leaf and pop in the oven for 90 minutes. Remove the bay leaf before serving.

Perfect served with mashed potato or pasta.

TOP TIP

Avoid bribery with food.
For example, try not to say things like 'if you don't eat this spinach you won't get any pudding'. Suggesting pudding's nicer than a main can further establish the perception that savoury food, and by its nature meat and veg, is not as tasty as something sweet.

SLOW-COOKED LAMB

This meltingly soft dish has been known to win over even the most reluctant carnivores – sometimes it is texture alone that puts a child off and this dish makes the meat easy to chew. It takes very little preparation but benefits from several hours in the oven, so a great one for weekends instead of a standard roast.

Ingredients:

3 tbsp cooking oil (vegetable or olive)

Half a leg of lamb (about 1¼ kg)

Seasoning (salt, if desired, and pepper)

4 large onions

300 ml red wine

Optional extras: Handful of thyme sprigs, large handful of parsley.

Preheat oven to 160°C/325°F/ gas mark 3.

Heat the olive oil in a large flameproof casserole dish, add the meat, season and fry on a fairly high heat for about 8 minutes, turning until it is evenly well browned. Remove and set aside.

Thinly slice the onions, add them to the pan and fry for about 10 minutes, until softened and slightly browned. Add a few of the thyme sprigs if using and cook for a further minute or so. Season if desired.

Sit the lamb on top of the onions, add the wine then cover and cook for 3 hours.

Serve with mashed potato and veg of your choice.

CORNED BEEF HASH

This surprisingly tasty wartime favourite deserves its place alongside our family-friendly main dishes, and what's more it's great value as well as nutritious.

Ingredients:

400 g potatoes

25 g butter

1 medium onion

1 tbsp cooking oil (vegetable or olive)

340 g tin of corned beef

Seasoning (salt, if desired, and pepper)

75 g Cheddar cheese

Preheat the oven to 180°C/350°F/ gas mark 4.

Peel and chop the potatoes, boil for 15 minutes or until soft and mash with butter. Peel and finely chop the onion, heat the oil in a medium-sized frying pan and gently fry until soft. Crumble the corned beef into a mixing bowl, add the fried onion, season and mix well. If you prefer, avoid 'bits' by using puréed onion or ice cube onion purée and miss out the frying stage (remember to defrost the purée). Transfer the mixture to an ovenproof dish and spread the mashed potato over the meat mixture.

Grate the cheese and sprinkle over the potato then bake for 30 minutes in the preheated oven.

COTTAGE PIE

Another comforting classic that should satisfy even the fussiest of eaters.

Ingredients:

1 medium onion

2 medium carrots

1 tbsp cooking oil (vegetable or olive)

500 g lean minced beef

1 x 400 g can of chopped tomatoes

300 ml beef stock

Seasoning (salt, if desired, and pepper)

750 g mashed potato

25 g butter

Optional: 1 tsp Worcestershire sauce. Really, this dish needs this glorious flavour but if your child struggles with any piquant taste it can be omitted.

Preheat the oven to 190°C/375°F/ gas mark 5.

Peel and finely chop the onion and carrots. Heat the oil in a large frying pan and add the onion and carrots. Fry for 5 minutes until they begin to soften. Add the beef and fry for a further 10 minutes until it browns – make sure you break the mince up to ensure even cooking. Stir occasionally. Pour in the tomatoes and stir in the stock and season. Bring the mixture to the boil, reduce the heat and simmer for 10 minutes. Add the Worcestershire sauce if desired.

Transfer the mixture to an ovenproof dish and evenly spread the mashed potato over the top. Bake in the preheated oven for 30 minutes.

MEATBALLS

Great on their own or added to a basic tomato sauce (see page 27) and served with your favourite pasta.

Ingredients:

3 slices bread (fresh or a few days old)

1 medium onion

500 g minced beef

1 egg

Seasoning (salt, if desired, and pepper)

2 tbsp olive oil

Optional extras: 1 tbsp of parsley; 1 tsp of smooth French mustard; 1 tsp chilli powder.

Remove the crusts from the bread, then tear into minuscule pieces. Those with a blender can give them a whizz for a few seconds.

Peel and chop the onion. Mix together with the breadcrumbs and add the mince, (and the optional chilli powder, mustard or chopped parsley leaves) beaten egg and seasoning, and mould into balls.

Heat the oil in a frying pan and fry the balls evenly for about 10–15 minutes, turning regularly. Don't make the balls too big or they will not cook in the middle.

PORK STIR-FRY

The pork really lifts the flavour of this dish, but you could try using other meats, such as chicken or beef.

Ingredients:

1 onion

1 clove of garlic

1 green pepper

1 red pepper

1 tbsp cooking oil (vegetable or olive)

1 tbsp soy sauce

250 g diced pork

Seasoning (salt, if desired, and pepper)

Optional: If peppers aren't popular then switch to other veg such as mangetout, peas or broccoli.

Peel and chop the onion and garlic, and chop and deseed the peppers. Heat the oil in a large frying pan or wok, then fry the onion and the garlic for about 3–4 minutes. Add the peppers, soy sauce and the pork and fry until the pork is cooked. This should take about 10 minutes, depending on the size of the meat pieces. Season and serve with rice or egg noodles.

SHEPHERD'S PIE

Another family favourite to comfort and enjoy. There are plenty of variations to this dish, but we reckon the original is the best.

Ingredients:

1 medium onion

750 g potatoes

25 g butter

2 tbsp milk

Seasoning (salt, if desired, and pepper)

2 tbsp cooking oil (vegtable or olive)

575 g cooked lamb, minced/or raw minced lamb

2 tbsp tomato purée

Dash of Worcestershire sauce

400 ml chicken or beef stock

Optional: For a little added luxury, grate Cheddar cheese over the mash before baking.

Preheat the oven to 180°C/350°F/ gas mark 4.

Peel and chop the onion and potatoes. Cook the potatoes in salted boiling water until soft. Drain the potatoes, then mash with the butter and milk, add salt and pepper to taste if required. Set aside.

Heat the oil in a large frying pan, add the onion and fry gently for 5 minutes. (If you're using raw minced lamb, add the meat to the frying pan and gently fry off for a further 5 minutes.)

Stir in the cooked minced lamb, tomato purée, Worcestershire sauce and seasoning if desired. Add the stock and bring to the boil. Then simmer for 5 minutes and transfer to a pie dish. Spoon the mash over the meat so that it's evenly covered and there are no gaps, and put in the oven. Bake for 20–25 minutes, or until the potatoes are browned.

SHISH KEBAB (LAMB)

The shish kebab as we know it today is a staple of the British takeaway scene, but home-made kebabs taste so much better and are often far healthier. This is another good dish to get the children to help prepare.

Ingredients:

375 g lamb (leg meat)

150 g natural yoghurt

Juice of 1 lemon

2 tbsp olive oil – 1 tbsp for frying, 1 tbsp for binding

Fresh rosemary for the marinade

Seasoning (salt, if desired, and pepper)

Optional: Add 1 tsp ground cumin to the yoghurt.

Prepare this meal well in advance, as the lamb has to marinate for at least a couple of hours in order to obtain its full flavour. Cut the lamb into small cubes and place in a bowl with the yoghurt, lemon juice, olive oil rosemary and seasoning (including cumin if desired). Stir well, then put the bowl in the fridge for a couple of hours, making sure the lamb is evenly coated in the marinade.

When ready to be cooked, soak four wooden skewers in water for a few minutes, then divide the meat onto them, place on the grill pan with the rosemary and grill for 10 to 15 minutes, turning the kebabs occasionally so they cook evenly. If there is any spare marinade use it to flavour the meat while it is being grilled.

Serve with salad and pitta bread.

STICKY RIBS

This delicious marinade will transform the ribs into a teatime treat the children will love. Don't be put off by the marinade ingredients; they all meld into a sticky coating that's sweet and tempting.

Ingredients:

1 kg small, lean pork ribs

For the marinade:

2 cloves of garlic

500 g carton of passata

2 tbsp soy sauce

3 tbsp honey

1 tbsp Worcestershire sauce

Preheat oven to 200°C/390°F/ gas mark 6.

Peel and crush the garlic. In a large bowl, mix together the passata, garlic, soy sauce, honey and Worcestershire sauce.

Add the pork ribs to the bowl and mix well to coat evenly. The easiest way is to use your fingers. Cover the bottom of a large roasting tin with foil as this will make it much easier to clean. Lay the ribs and all the sauce into the tin. Cover with foil and bake for 35 minutes.

Remove the foil cover from the tray and bake the ribs for a further 30–40 minutes, turning occasionally. If the ribs look like they are starting to burn, add a couple of tablespoons of water.

SWEET, SLOW-COOKED BELLY OF PORK

When standard roasts have defeated the younger family members, this one has been a hit. The secret is its super-slow cook, ensuring the meat is sweet, succulent and beautifully tender.

Ingredients:

1.5 kg piece pork belly, skin scored

2 tbsp olive oil

Seasoning (coarse sea salt and black pepper if desired)

Preheat oven to 180°C/350°F/gas mark 4.

Rub the oil all over the skin of the pork, and work some sea salt into the skin. Coarse sea salt creates a better crackling.

Place the pork, skin-side up, on a rack in a roasting tin. Cook for 1 hour. Remove from the oven and baste with the juices. Continue to cook for a further hour, basting every 20 minutes. Turn up the oven to 210°C/425°F/gas mark 7 and cook for a further 30–40 minutes, so you get perfect crackling. Once this has been achieved, leave to rest for 15 minutes.

Optional extras: The pork belly can be enhanced with flavours such as toasted fennel seeds, garlic, lemon and Chinese five spice.

TOP TIP

Remember that it takes at least seven times of tasting something new before reluctant taste buds can really decide whether they're prepared to go along with a new taste.

> When my children were younger they ate a wider variety of foods. As they approached school age they became fussier. The two older children, now in their twenties, have once again broadened their tastes, despite one being vegetarian.

MUM OF THREE, AGED 8, 20 AND 23

> Jake will eat anything for Aunty Jo, and will try different foods and eat them at his friend Simon's house.

JON, DAD OF JAKE, AGED 9

> We were told by a dietician that children have to try a food 20 times before they can decide whether they like it or not, so we always remind them of this and get them to try a little of what they don't like as many times as we can. Evie has developed a liking for more spiced foods and fish as a result.

TOAD IN THE HOLE

A real crowd-pleaser of a dish and simple to make.

Ingredients:

100 g flour

Seasoning (salt, if desired, and pepper)

1 egg

250 ml milk

500 g sausages

3 tbsp cooking oil (vegetable or olive)

Optional: To add even more flavour to this dish, try wrapping the sausages in thinly sliced pancetta, serrano ham or streaky bacon – a sort of pigs in blankets in the hole!

Preheat the oven to 200°C/390°F/ gas mark 6.

Place the flour in a bowl and mix in a pinch of salt if desired, then make a well and break the egg into it. Add first a little milk and mix together to give a smooth texture, then pour in the rest of the milk and beat for a minute or so to form a batter. Put the sausages in a baking tin with the oil and bake for 10 minutes. Then pour in the batter and cook for a further 25 minutes or until the batter has risen and is browned.

Serve with peas or freshly steamed green vegetables.

ROAST CHICKEN

It is important not to overcook chicken as it loses all its flavour and is harder to carve, yet it is imperative that the meat is fully cooked through. You can check by sticking a skewer or fork into the thigh of the bird, and if the juices run clear, it's good to eat.

Preheat oven to 180°C/350°F/ gas mark 4.

Place the chicken in a baking tin with 125 ml olive oil and season with plenty of black pepper and bake for 15–20 minutes per 500 g plus 20 minutes.

Options: There are numerous ways to enhance the chicken, such as sprinkling either dried or fresh herbs over the skin before cooking, coating the chicken with a honey and mustard glaze or putting two lemon halves in the cavity and dotting sliced cloves of garlic just under the skin.

TOP TIP

Don't let them fill up on drinks alone. Fussy eaters can often satisfy their hunger by drinking milk or fruit juice. Milk and juice are better served with a meal than between meals.

ROAST BEEF

Before throwing away the packaging for your joint, note how much it weighs. Allow 20 minutes cooking time per 500 g, plus 20 minutes on top – this will allow for cooking the meat 'English style', i.e. with not too much blood seeping out. If you prefer it 'rare', cook for about 15 minutes less.

Preheat oven to 180°C/350°F/ gas mark 4.

Put the joint in a roasting tin and pour 125 ml olive oil over the top and the sides. Season as desired and add any herbs of your choice, and pop into the oven.

The joint must be 'basted' – that means spooning the oil in the tin over the top of the meat to stop it from drying out. Repeat the basting process two or three times during cooking.

When the meat is cooked, carve the joint and serve with fresh vegetables and roast potatoes (see page 110). Gravy can be made from the juices in the roasting tin by adding a small amount of flour and stirring over a medium heat to thicken, then bulking up with more beef stock.

Roast beef has to be served with Yorkshire puddings (see page 111).

ROAST PORK

This must be cooked for a little longer than beef, as it is essential that pork is well cooked. Prepare in the same method as the beef but cook for 25 minutes per 500 g plus 25 minutes over, on the same oven setting. Baste the joint every 20 minutes. If you like garlic, try sticking whole cloves in the joint before cooking.

ROAST LAMB

Lamb has a wonderful flavour that makes it worth splashing out on occasionally.

Prepare in the same method as the beef and cook for 20 minutes per 500 g and 20 minutes extra on the same oven setting. Baste every 20 minutes.

Options: Add some sprigs of rosemary for extra flavour, and you can also dot slices of garlic into the flesh if you score the skin.

ROAST POTATOES

There's definitely a right way and a wrong way when it comes to cooking roasties, and here's the secret to lovely, fluffy potatoes that are golden and crunchy on the outside.

Ingredients:

1 kg floury potatoes, such as Maris Piper

Seasoning (salt, if desired, and pepper)

3 tbsp cooking oil (vegetable or olive)

Preheat the oven to 180°C/350°F/ gas mark 4.

Peel the potatoes and cut into large chunks. Parboil in boiling water (salted if desired) for about 5 minutes then drain and toss vigorously in the pan to roughen the edges.

Put a generous amount of cooking oil in a roasting tin and put in the oven, until smoking. Carefully take the tin out of the oven and add the potatoes to the hot fat, basting them as you do so.

Put the tin back in the oven and cook for about 1 hour until the roast potatoes are golden and crunchy on the outside and soft in the middle. Turn them over from time to time to make sure they colour on all sides.

YORKSHIRE PUDDING

A food marriage made in heaven when eaten with roast beef, but works equally well with any roast, including a nut roast.

Ingredients:

3 eggs

115 g flour

Seasoning to taste (salt, if desired, and pepper)

275 ml milk

2–3 tbsp cooking oil (vegetable)

Preheat the oven to 240°C/450°F/ gas mark 8.

Mix together the eggs and flour, with a pinch of salt and pepper if desired.

Add the milk, gently whisking until you have a runny batter.

Cover and leave this to rest in the fridge for up to 12 hours, but try to let it stand for at least 20 minutes to reach room temperature before using.

Drizzle a little oil in the bottom of each of the compartments of a 12-hole muffin tray, or if you are using a rectangular roasting tray, cover the bottom of the tray.

Heat the oil in the oven for about 5 minutes, until it is piping hot.

Remove the roasting tray from the oven, pour in the batter, and immediately return to the oven. Bake for 25 minutes, until golden brown and crispy, making sure not to open the oven door for the first 20 minutes, if you want to avoid your pudding losing its puffed up appearance!

CAULIFLOWER CHEESE

A quick and cheap dish that can be prepared with ease. Makes a great accompaniment to roast beef or pork.

Ingredients:

50 g butter

50 g cornflour

375 ml milk

150 g Cheddar cheese

Seasoning (salt, if desired, and pepper)

1 cauliflower

Prepare the cheese sauce as outlined in the sauces section, page 26, (using 100 g of the cheese) but use 375 ml milk instead of 500 ml, and add seasoning. Break the cauliflower into florets then place in boiling water for about 10 minutes, making sure it is not overcooked.

When the cauliflower is cooked, drain well and place in an ovenproof dish, pour over the cheese sauce, sprinkle on the remaining 50 g of grated cheese and brown under a hot grill.

CHEESY POTATO PIE

Comfort food, comfort food, comfort food – need we say more.

Ingredients:

175 g Cheddar cheese

1 medium onion

1.5 kg potatoes

2 tbsp butter

1 tbsp milk

Preheat oven to 180°C/ 350°F/ gas mark 4.

Grate the cheese. Peel and dice the onion and potatoes and bring to the boil in a large pan. Once soft, drain and mash the potato with butter and milk, gradually add two thirds of the cheese until well mixed.

Transfer the mixture to an ovenproof dish, cover with the remaining cheese and bake until the cheese has melted and started to brown. This dish can be served with any variety of in-season steamed vegetables.

EGG FRIED RICE

This incredibly simple dish is a great way of providing protein and carbs together, and if you serve it with the optional vegetables or some chopped raw pepper you have a lovely balanced dish.

Ingredients:

300 g long grain rice

Seasoning (salt, if desired, and pepper)

2 large eggs

2 tbsp cooking oil (vegetable)

Soy sauce

Optional extras: 100 g frozen peas; 100 g canned or frozen sweetcorn.

Bring three pints of water to boil in a large pan, add the rice and salt if desired, bring back to the boil and cook for 12 minutes, until tender. Drain well, rinse with cold water and leave for 15–20 minutes to drain thoroughly in a colander.

Beat the eggs and set aside. Heat the oil in a large frying pan or wok and add the cold cooked rice and any optional extras and stir-fry over a medium-high heat for a further 2–3 minutes.

Add the egg and stir everything together until the eggs have set. Season with soy sauce and black pepper, then serve.

VEGETABLE KEBAB

This recipe can be adjusted to suit your child's tastes, by using more or fewer of the ingredients depending on what is palatable.

Ingredients:

1 small onion

1 pepper

1 courgette

2 tomatoes

4 mushrooms

25 g butter

Seasoning (salt, if desired, and pepper)

Soak a couple of wooden skewers in water for a few minutes. Meanwhile, peel the onion and deseed the pepper, then cut all the vegetables into large chunks, or quarters. Soften the butter. Thread all the vegetables onto the water-soaked skewers and daub them with butter. Place under a medium grill for about 15 minutes. Season if desired.

Optional: To pep up this recipe try adding different flavours according to taste, such as a sprinkle of soy sauce, pesto, honey, etc. before grilling or barbecuing.

VEGETABLE STIR-FRY

This dish is not only healthy, but is remarkably tasty and surprisingly filling with the bonus of being meat-free for children who dislike the texture, taste or smell of meat. It offers a range of new textures without overwhelming the taste buds with strong flavours.

Ingredients:

1 medium onion

1 clove of garlic

1 medium carrot

1 red pepper

1 green pepper

2 tbsp cooking oil (vegetable or olive)

1 x tin of water chestnuts

1 x tin of bamboo shoots

2 tbsp soy sauce

Seasoning (salt, if desired, and pepper)

1 pack of fresh beansprouts

Prepare all the vegetables first: peel and chop the onion, garlic and carrot, and chop and deseed the red and green peppers. Pour the oil into your wok or frying pan over a high heat, then when it is smoking add the onion and garlic, and fry for 5 minutes, stirring constantly. If you are using water chestnuts, cook these first as they take the longest to cook and are nicer when they are slightly crispy. Then add the soy sauce, seasoning and other vegetables except for the beansprouts if using.

After frying the vegetables for about 5–10 minutes, add the beansprouts and cook for a couple more minutes. It is important to keep the beansprouts firm. Serve with rice or noodles.

VEGETARIAN LASAGNE

The wonderful Mediterranean aroma of this dish as it cooks will get even the most reluctant of taste buds tingling – if your child is not a meat eater, this vegetarian option of a classic dish is a winner.

Ingredients:

1 large onion

1 clove of garlic

2 tbsp cooking oil (vegetable or olive)

1 medium leek

1 red pepper

1 green pepper

2 courgettes

1 x 400 g tin of chopped tomatoes

2 tbsp tomato purée

2 tsp oregano

Seasoning (salt, if desired, and pepper)

1 packet of lasagne ('no pre-cooking required' type)

Preheat oven to 200°C/350°F/ gas mark 6.

Peel and chop the onion and garlic, and cook with the oil in a large saucepan for 5 minutes. Then wash, trim and chop the leek, deseed the peppers and chop with the courgettes and add to the pan, frying gently for another 3 minutes or so. Or use the onion purée option on p.21. Then add the tomatoes, purée, oregano and seasoning, bring to the boil then simmer for a further 20 minutes. While the vegetable sauce is simmering prepare the cheese sauce. See instructions on page 26 for how to prepare the cheese sauce.

Grease a shallow baking dish, then add a layer of vegetable sauce, a layer of lasagne, a layer of cheese sauce, a layer of vegetable sauce, and so on, making sure to end up with cheese sauce on top. Then sprinkle on the remaining grated cheese. Bake for around 25 minutes.

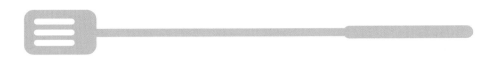

"

One of our children refused to eat anything besides yoghurt, puréed foods and milk between the age of 6 months and 3 years. We persevered with the 'keep trying a little each time' method and now she's the best eater ever. She even gets excited about trying new foods. The pain of fussy eating doesn't last forever but it seems endless at the time.

"

AMANDA, MOTHER OF EVIE AND CHLOE, AGED 6 AND 9

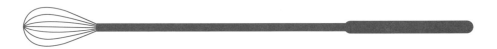

"

We have a rule in our house where the kids are not allowed to say they don't like a certain food. I don't expect them to finish everything on their plate but they must eat some of it... otherwise I'll make it for them every day! "

DANIELLE, MUM OF OLIVER AND SISSY, AGED 10 AND 7

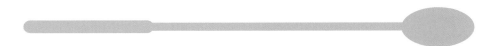

VEGGIE BURGERS

Burgers are such a good way of packing loads of goodness into one single parcel. This veggie option does just that and can be a great finger food for fun mealtimes.

Ingredients:

1 large onion

1 clove of garlic

2 medium carrots

2 medium courgettes

3 tbsp cooking oil (vegetable or olive) – 2 tbsp for binding, 1 tbsp for frying

1 tsp ground cumin

1 tsp ground coriander

2 tbsp chopped fresh coriander

Seasoning (salt, if desired, and pepper)

1 egg

100 g breadcrumbs

Peel and chop the onion and garlic, and coarsely grate the carrots and courgettes.

Heat the oil in a large frying pan, add the onion and garlic, and gently fry for 5 minutes, stirring frequently, until the onion is soft and beginning to brown. Add the carrots and courgettes, and fry for a further 10 minutes, stirring, until the vegetables have softened. Stir in the ground cumin and coriander, fresh coriander and seasoning to taste, and mix well. Remove the pan from the heat and set aside to cool slightly.

Beat the egg in a large bowl and mix all the vegetables into the bowl with the breadcrumbs until all ingredients are thoroughly combined, then shape the mixture into four thick burgers about 10 cm in diameter.

Heat the remaining oil in the now empty frying pan and gently fry the burgers for about 5 minutes on each side, or until they are firm and golden.

SNACKS AND LIGHT BITES

CRUNCHY VEGETABLES WITH SUNDRIED TOMATO DIP

Sometimes going back to basics is the best way of getting children to eat a range of vegetables. The riot of colours provided in this plateful of fresh vegetables is very appealing to children. The range of vegetable choice can be tempered to suit your child.

Ingredients:

1 x 200 g packet of soft cheese with garlic and herbs

100 g sundried tomatoes

30 ml oil from the jar of sundried tomatoes

180 g carrots

½ red pepper

½ yellow pepper

½ green pepper

2 celery sticks

100 g sugar snap peas

150 g cherry tomatoes

100 g cucumber

Blitz the soft cheese, sundried tomatoes and oil with a hand blender for 2–3 minutes until smooth.

Peel the carrots, core and deseed the peppers then cut each of the vegetables into strips. (It's best to cut the sugar snap peas in half lengthways and slice the cucumber into batons.)

Spoon the sundried tomato dip into a bowl and serve alongside the vegetables.

TOP TIP

Although we'd all like our children to eat nicely with a knife and fork, there's something to be said for finger food. Getting a child to touch and feel the texture of their food can help with the familiarisation process of making a child feel at ease with food.

BAKED POTATO (AND FILLINGS)

A crispy skin, lovely light fluffy centre and a fabulous filling makes for a delicious and nutritious meal.

Ingredients:

1 baking potato such as King Edward (judge the size according to appetite)

Filling of your choice

Suggestions for fillings:

Baked beans and tuna

Baked beans with Worcestershire sauce and a fried egg

Chilli and cheese

Coleslaw

Cottage cheese and chives

Pesto (see recipe for pesto on page 27)

Tuna and mayonnaise

After stabbing your potato several times with a sharp implement (preferably a fork) to pierce the skin, place in the oven for about 60 minutes: 210°C/425°F/gas mark 7.

Test the potato with a skewer or a knife to see if it is cooked in the middle. For a crispier skin, drizzle a little oil and salt over the potato and wrap in silver foil before putting it in the oven. For garlic fans, an interesting alternative is to mix some finely chopped garlic with butter and dollop this inside the potato halfway through cooking, then wrap in foil to contain the juices for the remainder of the cooking time.

CIABATTA PIZZA

Ring the changes with this slight variation on the standard and much loved pizza.

Ingredients:

1 ciabatta bread, cut in half lengthways

2 tomatoes, chopped

100 g grated cheese

12–15 slices salami or pepperoni

Seasoning (salt, if desired, and pepper)

Preheat the oven to 180°C/390°F/ gas mark 4.

Place the ciabatta halves on a baking tray. Divide the chopped tomatoes between the two halves and spread evenly. Then add half of the cheese, and the salami or pepperoni. Season then top with the remaining cheese.

Bake for 10–15 minutes until golden brown and the cheese is bubbling.

TOP TIP

Try different ways of eating – experiment with more unusual finger food such as sticky rice balls dipped in sauce, dabble with chopsticks, twizzle spaghetti…

CROQUE-MONSIEUR

This is simply delicious, albeit not the healthiest of choices. Maybe save it for a special occasion or when a bit of a treat is due!

Ingredients:

4 slices of bread (wholemeal or white depending on your tastes)

2 tsp mustard (Dijon is best)

80 g grated cheese (again, for an authentic French taste, try Gruyère)

2 slices ham

30 g butter

Preheat the oven to 180°C/350°F/ gas mark 4.

Spread half a teaspoon of mustard over each slice of bread, and then top two slices with layers of half of the grated cheese, followed by a slice of ham, and then the remaining cheese. Place the remaining two slices on top of the fillings to make a sandwich.

Heat butter in a large frying pan until sizzling, then place whole sandwiches in pan and fry for 1–2 minutes on each side until golden brown

Transfer sandwiches to a baking tray and place in the oven for 4–5 minutes, until cheese has melted.

Remove from oven, slice each sandwich in half and serve.

CROSTINI

You can choose virtually any topping you like for your crostini. Here is a classic and colourful combo.

Ingredients:

Base:

1 baguette

2 tbsp olive oil

1 clove of garlic

Topping:

2 large ripe tomatoes

2 tbsp olive oil

1 handful basil leaves

Seasoning (salt, if desired, and pepper)

Preheat the oven to 190°C/375°F/ gas mark 5.

Chop the tomatoes and place in a small bowl and mix with the oil, rip up the basil leaves and mix with the tomatoes. Season if desired.

Cut the baguette into slices and place on a large baking sheet, brush with oil and bake for 5 minutes to create the crostini base.

Remove the crostini from the oven. Cut the garlic clove in half and rub over the crostini then spoon the tomato mixture on top.

EGGY BREAD

A quick and easy light bite that everyone can enjoy.

Ingredients:

2 eggs

1 tbsp whole milk

Seasoning (salt, if desired, and pepper)

2 slices of bread

1 tbsp cooking oil (vegetable or olive)

Break the eggs into a bowl and beat them lightly, stir in the milk. Season if desired. Slice the bread into halves. Heat the oil in a frying pan. Dip the bread into the egg, then place the bread into the frying pan. Fry until both sides are golden brown. Remove from the pan and serve immediately.

TOP TIP

Limit snacks where you can, and only offer water with them to avoid your child decreasing his or her appetite for meals.

GARLIC BREAD

Get the kids to help prepare this and they'll enjoy it all the more.

Ingredients:

150 g butter

2 cloves of garlic

1 stick of French bread

Optional extra: Finely chopped parsley.

Preheat the oven to 190°C/375°F/gas mark 5. Put the butter in a small mixing bowl. It helps if the butter is soft. Peel and finely chop the garlic and add to the butter, mixing well with a fork (add parsley if using).

Cut into the French stick at 4 cm intervals, without actually slicing through it, and spread some of the butter on both sides of each slit. Then close up the gaps and wrap the loaf in foil. Place in the oven and cook for 15–20 minutes.

GUACAMOLE

Avocados are nutritional powerhouses, packed with healthy fats, protein, vitamins and minerals and dietary fibre, so give your kids the health benefits with this delicious dip.

Ingredients:

2 avocados

1 small red onion

1 clove garlic

1 ripe tomato

1 lime

Seasoning (salt, if desired, and pepper to taste)

Peel, stone and chop the avocados; peel and finely chop the onion and garlic; finely chop the tomato; juice the lime.

Mash avocados in a medium serving bowl. Stir in onion, garlic, tomato and lime juice. Season with salt and pepper to taste.

Serve as a dip with chopped raw vegetables such as cucumber, peppers, carrots, or simply dip breadsticks.

HUMMUS

Although hummus is available ready-made, it is cheaper to make your own. It's easier to use canned chick peas instead of soaking dried ones for hours. Note that a blender is needed for this recipe.

Ingredients:

2 cloves of garlic

2 tbsp cooking oil (vegetable or olive)

1 x 400 g can of chickpeas

Juice of 1 lemon

100 g natural unsweetened yoghurt

½ tsp ground cumin

Peel and chop the garlic. Put all the ingredients in a blender and blitz until a soft consistency is achieved. Then put in a dish and place in the fridge to chill for an hour or two.

Chop some raw vegetables such as carrots, cucumber, red pepper or slice some pitta bread for dipping into this delicious garlicky concoction.

TOP TIP

Research shows that repeated exposure to new tastes can increase the chances of a child learning to like a food.

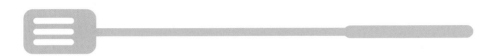

" I've found that introducing a variety of foods from the start makes them more accepting of different flavours. From a young age we'd let them try little bits of spicy food until they got used to it so now they've grown to accept it. "

PENNY, MUM OF LAUREN AND CHARLIE,
AGED 13 AND 10

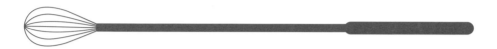

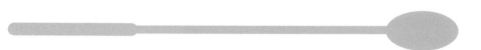

"
I do believe that parents have a great influence over their children's tastes – if they are fussy eaters themselves then their children will probably be fussy too. If the parents don't like a certain food they are unlikely to prepare it for their children.
"

LUCY, MUM OF MIA AND LUKE, AGED 9 AND 6

OMELETTE

A really easy way to use up eggs, or knock together a quick and filling snack.

Ingredients:

2 or 3 eggs

Seasoning (salt, if desired, and pepper)

25 g butter

Optional extra: Pinch of mixed herbs.

Beat the eggs together in a mixing bowl and add the seasoning (and herbs if using). Melt the butter in a frying pan and pour in the eggs.

As soon as the eggs start to cook, lift up one edge of the omelette with a spatula, tilt the pan and let the uncooked egg run underneath. Continue to do this until the omelette is cooked, then flip it in half and serve on a warmed plate.

To add interest, you could try one of these variations:

Cheese and tomato
Prepare as above, but add 50 g grated cheese and 1 chopped tomato before pouring into the frying pan.

Bacon
Cut 2 rashers of bacon up into little pieces and fry for a couple of minutes, then add to the mixture and follow the instructions above.

OPEN SANDWICHES

An open sandwich is, quite simply, a sandwich without a top slice of bread which makes it less filling for smaller appetites, and means that knives and forks have to come into play unless you want to get really messy eating them. Any of the following make great toppings but use your imagination to match the tastes of your child:

Cream cheese with sliced tomatoes or grapes

Smoked salmon with cream cheese (and cucumber if your child likes it)

Peanut butter (go on, add some jam if you like!)

Hummus, with finely chopped red pepper if tastes allow (see page 131 for hummus recipe)

Tuna mixed with a couple of spoonfuls of mayonnaise and some chopped cucumber

PIZZA

There is huge scope for variety here, both in toppings and bases, so don't be afraid to experiment! The easiest to make is the French bread pizza, because the base is simply a sliced baguette. Dough bases can be bought ready-made, but they cost more than French sticks or home-made dough.

PIZZA MARGHERITA

This is the basic pizza. If you want to design your own, use this and add your own toppings. To add a touch of authenticity, sprinkle some basil on top – the mozzarella, tomato and basil recreate the colours of the Italian flag.

Ingredients:

1 stick of French bread

2 tbsp tomato purée

50 g mozzarella cheese

Pepper

Pinch of oregano

1 tsp cooking oil (vegetable or olive)

Slice the French stick in half and spread some tomato purée on top. A thin layer will do – if you put too much on your pizza it will become soggy. Place slices of cheese on top, season, add the oregano (and basil if desired) and pour on the oil. Bake in the oven until the cheese turns a golden brown colour. It should take roughly 15 minutes at 210 °C/425 °F/gas mark 7. If you don't like/can't afford mozzarella, ordinary Cheddar cheese does the trick.

QUICHE LORRAINE

Eggs aren't to every child's taste but, sometimes, miraculously, when they're disguised in this recipe they become palatable – at least that's what we've found.

Ingredients for shortcrust pastry:

200 g plain flour

100 g butter

3 tbsp water

Pinch of salt (if desired)

Ingredients for filling:

100 g bacon

4 eggs

250 ml milk

Seasoning (salt, if desired, and pepper)

Optional: 50 g cheese.

This is perhaps one of the only times when it's worth sieving the flour (and salt if using), but don't worry if you don't have a sieve. Keep the butter cold and cut into cubes, add to the flour and start rubbing with your fingertips.

After rubbing in, add some water a little at a time. The water is needed to bind the mixture together, but be careful not to add so much as to make the pastry become sticky. Mould the pastry into a ball then roll out on a floured board or very clean floured work surface. Also sprinkle a coating of flour onto the rolling pin (you can always improvise with a wine bottle if you don't have a rolling pin). The flour is used to stop the pastry from sticking to the board and the pin.

Roll the pastry so that its area is big enough to cover the flan dish, then carefully place the pastry over the dish and mould it in the shape of the dish. Remove the edge of the overlapping pastry by running a knife along the rim of the dish.

Cut the bacon into small pieces, then fry lightly for a couple of minutes and place on the bottom of the pastry base. Beat the eggs together, add the milk, season and beat again.

Pour over the bacon, grate the cheese and sprinkle on top if desired and bake in a hot oven at 200°C/390°F/ gas mark 6 for 25 minutes or until the filling has set.

TOP TIP

Get creative: design a picture on the plate – mashed-potato hair, peas for eyes, a carrot nose, a sausage smile, or create patterns on the plate to make food look more interesting.

PITTAS AND WRAPS

Pittas and wraps are a popular choice for children as an alternative to sandwiches as they can be easier to eat than big chunks of bread. Pittas are great either sliced for dipping or cut them in half to create two pockets for filling. Wraps speak for themselves.

Filling suggestions:

Grated cheese mixed with cream cheese

Tuna mayonnaise with sweetcorn

Cream cheese with ham or smoked salmon

Mozzarella, tomato and pesto

Grated carrot with sultanas and mayonnaise

Peanut butter and jam

Mashed banana with Nutella

COOKIES AND CAKES

BANANA BREAD

Many children (and adults too) find the look and taste of an overripe banana off-putting. Don't waste them though, they're perfect for use in this recipe.

Ingredients:

4 small ripe bananas

110 g butter

225 g caster sugar

2 eggs

90 ml milk

1 tsp vanilla extract

275 g plain flour

1 tsp bicarbonate of soda

Preheat the oven to 180°C/350°F/ gas mark 4. Grease a 20 cm x 12.5 cm loaf tin.

Mash the bananas.

In a large mixing bowl, beat together the butter and sugar until light and fluffy. Beat the eggs then add the bananas, milk and vanilla extract, and stir well.

Sift in the flour and bicarbonate of soda and fold the mixture until combined.

Transfer the mixture to the loaf tin and bake for 55–60 minutes, or until golden brown.

CARROT CAKE

This is a great way of sneaking a vegetable into a sweet thing and, unless you tell them they're there, children don't even notice the carrots.

Ingredients:

For the cake:

250 g carrots

200 g plain flour

2 tsp baking powder

1 tsp salt

1 tsp bicarbonate of soda

200 g brown sugar

150 ml vegetable oil

2 eggs

Optional: 110 g walnuts. These add a lovely crunch to the texture of this cake but if 'bits' are a deal-breaker they can be omitted.

For the icing:

110 g butter

225 g cream cheese

50g icing sugar

1 tsp vanilla extract

Preheat the oven to 160°C/325°F/gas mark 3. Grease a 23 cm cake tin.

Peel and grate the carrots.

In a large bowl, sift the flour, baking powder, salt and bicarbonate of soda and stir well. Add the sugar, carrot, walnuts, oil and beaten eggs, and stir until combined. Transfer to the tin, and bake for 65–70 minutes.

Place on a wire rack and allow to cool before removing from the cake tin.

In a small bowl, beat together the butter and cream cheese until light and fluffy. Add the sugar and vanilla extract and stir well. Spread the icing over the cake using a palette knife

142

CHOCOLATE BROWNIES

Sticky, gooey, fudgy – who doesn't love a brownie. This simple recipe will have them asking for more as soon as this batch is demolished.

Ingredients:

150 g unsalted butter

200 g dark chocolate

2 eggs

200 g dark muscovado sugar

100 g plain flour

1 tsp baking powder

Grease an 18 cm square cake tin with a little of the butter and line with non-stick baking parchment (or greaseproof paper). Break the chocolate into pieces and place with the butter in a heatproof bowl over a pan of simmering water. Don't let the water boil, or else the water will spill over.

Stir the chocolate and butter mixture together with a spoon. Beat the eggs and sugar together in a separate bowl using a handheld mixer if you have one, or by hand if you don't. Add in the melted chocolate and butter, and then the flour and baking powder. Stir thoroughly.

Pour the mixture into the tin and bake in a pre-heated oven for 30 minutes, at 160°C/325°F/gas mark 3. Allow to cool for 10 minutes before cutting into squares.

CHOCOLATE CHIP COOKIES

This lovely, simple recipe is a great one to cook with your children. They'll love getting involved and they'll love the results even more. Don't forget to let these treats cool before they're eaten… if you can!

Ingredients:

75 g butter

75 g granulated sugar

25 g brown sugar

1 egg

2 drops vanilla essence

100 g cooking chocolate

150 g self-raising flour

Grease a flat baking tray with a knob of butter. Cream the butter and the sugars either in a mixer or with a wooden spoon. Beat in the egg and vanilla. Grate or chop the chocolate coarsely, then stir into the creamed mixture along with the flour. Using a teaspoon place balls of the mixture on the baking tray, spaced well apart as they spread as they cook. Bake in the centre of a pre-heated oven for about 15 minutes at 190°C/375°F/gas mark 5. Place on a wire tray and leave until cold.

TOP TIP

Try some baking together. Get them to help out with straightforward tasks such as weighing out ingredients, sifting some flour, breaking an egg, beating a batter or rolling some dough.

CHOCOLATE CRISPY CAKES

Nothing could be simpler than this old favourite that takes barely any cooking. It's a perfect Easter recipe if you add some chocolate eggs to the 'nests'.

Ingredients:

50 g butter

4 tbsp golden syrup

100 g dark chocolate

75 g cornflakes

Gently melt the butter, syrup and chocolate in an oven-proof bowl over a bain-marie (place water in a pan, place oven-proof bowl over pan, making sure the bowl does not touch the water, then bring the water to the boil and simmer until the contents of the bowl melt, then stir together until smooth). Remove the bowl from the heat then stir in the cornflakes.

Place spoonfuls of the mixture into individual paper cupcake holders in a cupcake baking tin and leave to set in the refrigerator.

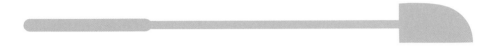

" I think a lot of the time we make our children's choices too easy. My parents said, 'This is what's for dinner, eat it or be hungry.' I am not a fussy eater! "

GEOFF, DAD OF TWO, AGED 5 AND 7

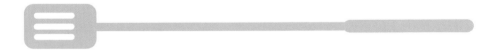

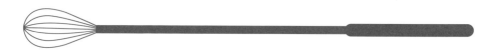

"

My daughter has difficulty using everyday cutlery so meat has to be prepared so that she can use her adaptable cutlery and crockery. Risotto is excellent for including new vegetables. It takes a long time for her to eat so her sister and I have to be patient. "

CHERYL, MUM OF TWINS, CHARLOTTE
AND FLORENCE, AGED 6

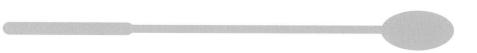

CHOCOLATE FRIDGE CAKE

Another fabulous chocolatey treat that, like the crispy cakes, requires virtually no cooking, making it a great recipe for children to help with.

Ingredients:

100 g dried apricots

250 g digestive biscuits

150 g milk chocolate

150 g dark chocolate

100 g unsalted butter

150 g golden syrup

75 g raisins

Melt the chocolate, butter and golden syrup in a bain-marie (place water in a pan, place oven-proof bowl over pan, making sure the bowl does not touch the water, then bring the water to the boil and simmer until the contents of the bowl melt, then stir together until smooth).

Remove the bowl from the heat and stir in the broken biscuits, apricots and raisins.

Spoon the mixture into the tin and press down until the surface is even.

Leave to cool, then put the chocolate mixture in the fridge for 1–2 hours to set.

Finely chop the apricots. Line a 20 cm square shallow container with cling film, leaving extra cling film hanging over the sides.

Put the biscuits into a plastic bag and crush them into pieces using a rolling pin.

Once the cake is hard, remove from the container and peel off the cling film then cut the cake into squares.

CUPCAKES

No birthday party is complete without cupcakes but these sweet treats can be made at any time of year – eat them plain or decorate them according to season: chocolate eggs at Easter, spooky iced faces for Halloween, red icing with silver balls at Christmas – use your imagination.

Ingredients:

For the cakes:

110 g butter

110 g caster sugar

2 eggs

1 tsp vanilla extract

110 g self-raising flour

2 tbsp milk

For the buttercream icing:

75 g unsalted butter

2 tbsp milk

1 tsp vanilla extract

225 g icing sugar

Preheat the oven to 180°C/350°F/gas mark 4. Line two 12-hole fairy cake tins with paper cases.

In a large bowl, beat together the butter (softened butter works best) and sugar until light and fluffy. Gradually add the eggs and vanilla extract, and beat until combined. Sift in the flour and fold the mixture to combine, then stir in the milk. Half-fill each case with the mixture, and bake for 10 minutes, or until golden brown. Place on a wire rack and allow to cool.

For the buttercream icing, mix 140 g of softened butter with 280 g of icing sugar and a tsp of milk and have fun decorating.

FLAPJACKS

The buttery loveliness of this traditional recipe makes for a wonderful recipe – yes, it's full of sugar too, but there are some healthy oats in the mix and it you spare this as a treat...

Ingredients:

175 g butter

175 g muscovado sugar

175 g golden syrup

340 g porridge oats

Preheat the oven to 150°C/300°F/ gas mark 2. Grease a 20 cm square baking tin and line with baking paper.

Melt the butter in a small pan over a low heat, then gradually add the sugar and syrup and stir until the sugar is dissolved.

Remove from the heat, then add in the porridge oats and mix well.

Transfer the mixture to the baking tin and use a wooden spoon to compact.

Bake for 40 minutes and allow to cool before cutting into squares or slices.

GINGERBREAD MEN

This is a great recipe to make with children – have fun with the cutter shapes as you can replace men with stars, chickens, circles... you name it – even have a go at icing decorations if you fancy it.

Ingredients:

340 g plain flour

1 tsp bicarbonate of soda

1 tsp ground cinnamon

2 tsp ground ginger

110 g butter

175 g light brown sugar

1 egg

4 tbsp golden syrup

Preheat the oven to 180°C/350°F/gas mark 4. Line a baking tray with baking paper.

Sift the flour into a bowl, add the bicarbonate of soda, cinnamon and ginger, and stir.

Beat in the butter and sugar.

In a separate bowl, beat the egg with the golden syrup, then add this to the mixture until it forms a dough.

Knead the dough on a lightly floured work surface until smooth, then wrap in cling film and chill in the fridge for 20 minutes.

Roll out the dough and cut out the gingerbread men with a cutter. Place them on the baking tray, leaving about 5 cm between each biscuit.

Bake for 15 minutes, or until golden brown.

JAM BUNS

Gooey jam adds that special dimension to these bite-sized treats – make sure they're cool enough to eat though!

Ingredients:

110 g butter

200 g self-raising flour

110 g caster sugar

1 egg (medium)

1 tbsp of milk

12 tsp of jam

Preheat the oven to 180°C/350°F/ gas mark 4.

Keep the butter cold and chop into cubes. Sieve the flour into a bowl then rub the butter into the flour with your fingers until it looks like breadcrumbs. Stir in the sugar.

Break the egg into a bowl and add the milk. Whisk together. Add the egg and milk mixture to the bowl with the flour, butter and sugar then knead the mixture until fully combined in the form of a firm ball.

Cut the ball into 12 equal pieces, rolling each to form further balls. Put the balls on to a baking sheet lined with greaseproof paper and squash each one down slightly.

Make a well in each ball by pressing your thumb down in the centre and fill with a teaspoon of jam.

Bake the buns for about 10–12 minutes.

Leave to cool thoroughly before eating.

JAM TARTS

'The Queen of Hearts' loves these jewel-like confections. Cheery to the last, you can make a treasure chest of colours, depending on the jam you use.

Ingredients:

75 g butter

150 g plain flour

Pinch of salt

50 g caster sugar

1 egg yolk

1 tbsp cold water

Jam of your choice

Preheat the oven to 190°C/375°F/gas mark 5. Grease a 12–16-hole tart tray.

Keep the butter cold and chop into cubes. Sieve the flour and salt into a bowl then rub the butter into the flour with your fingers until it looks like breadcrumbs. Add the sugar and egg yolk and stir well. Add water if necessary to form a dough.

Knead the dough gently, then wrap in cling film and chill in the fridge for 15 minutes.

On a lightly floured work surface, roll out the pastry to a ½ cm thickness. Cut into rounds to slightly overfill the holes in the tray, and press one into each hole.

Put spoonfuls of jam into each pastry case, making sure they are not overfilled.

Bake for 15–18 minutes, or until golden brown.

MILLIONAIRE SHORTBREAD

The rich quality of this treat gives the recipe its name – buttery biscuit base, gooey caramel middle and luxurious chocolate topping – who can refuse one?

Ingredients:

For the shortbread:

175 g butter

225 g plain flour

75 g caster sugar

2 tsp vanilla essence

For the caramel:

200 g butter

400 g condensed milk

4 tbsp golden syrup

1 tsp salt (if desired)

For the topping:

340 g milk chocolate

Preheat the oven to 180°C/350°F/gas mark 4. Grease a 20 cm square cake tin and line with baking paper.

Keep the butter cold and chop into cubes. Sieve the flour into a bowl then rub the butter into the flour with your fingers until it looks like breadcrumbs. Add the sugar and vanilla essence and stir well to form a rough dough. Transfer to the cake tin and press down to compact. Bake for 40 minutes, reducing the heat of the oven to 150°C/300°F/gas mark 2 after 10 minutes. Allow to cool in the tin.

In a large saucepan, bring the butter, condensed milk, syrup and salt (if using) to the boil and simmer for 10 minutes. Pour the mixture over the shortbread, then chill in the fridge for 30 minutes until hardened.

Gently melt the chocolate in a heatproof bowl over a pan of boiling water. Pour the chocolate over the caramel and chill in the fridge for a further 30 minutes, or until set. Cut into squares.

SHORTBREAD

The wonderfully buttery nature of these biscuits makes them a tempting treat throughout the year and it's a great recipe to try out with children as there's very little that can go wrong.

Ingredients:

225 g plain flour

40 g icing sugar

175 g butter

Preheat the oven to 180°C/350°F/ gas mark 4.

Sift the flour and icing sugar into a bowl and rub the butter in until it's well blended. Roll out the dough to the approximate thickness of a thumbnail and cut into it with 5 cm circular pastry cutters.

Transfer pastry rounds to a flat baking tin lined with greaseproof paper, place into the oven and bake for 15–20 minutes until they begin to brown and are firm to the touch.

TOP TIP

Persevere with different textures – it's tempting to purée stuff because that's what toddlers are brought up on so it's what they are used to but, the longer you keep to purées, the more difficult it will be to transition to different textures.

PUDDINGS

AVOCADO CHOCOLATE MOUSSE

'Avocado?' we hear you cry – yes, an unlikely coupling with chocolate but you'll never really know there's a green thing hiding in this great dessert.

Ingredients:

2 ripe avocados

1 tbsp unsweetened cocoa powder

1 heaped tbsp honey

1 tbsp cold water

Split the avocados and take out the large pips then spoon out the flesh into a bowl. Add the cocoa, honey and water and blitz with a hand blender until smooth. Chill until you're ready to serve.

TOP TIP

Invite them to smell and taste things along the way to help engage them in the activity. Often they'll be more willing to try something when they've helped to make it.

BAKED APPLES

Simple and wholesome, these winter warmers are a lovely, light end to a meal.

Ingredients (per apple):

Cooking apples (cater according to appetite)

2 tsp dried fruit (sultanas, raisins, currants)

1 tsp honey

Wash and core the apple and place on a piece of foil that will easily wrap around the apple.

Combine honey with dried fruit then fill the cavity in the apple.

Wrap the apple with the remaining foil.

Bake the foil-wrapped apple for 45 minutes in a preheated oven at 200°C/390°F/gas mark 6.

Remove from oven, remove foil, allow to cool and serve with natural yoghurt or cream.

159

> "Charlotte enjoys cooking and this helps her to consider new foods.

> "Noah will eat cheese if it's melted or cooked in a sauce but not in its original state. He maintains that he dislikes cheese but has not actually tried it for a long time.

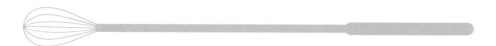

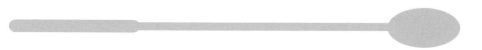

"We've always encouraged Jane to try foods even when she has refused them. The phrase in our house is 'you can't say you don't like something until you've tried it!' We feel this approach works."

BARBECUED BANANA WITH CHOCOLATE

This quick and easy dessert is a favourite for barbecues.

Ingredients:

Milk or dark chocolate

Banana

Break the chocolate into small chunks. Do not peel the banana, instead, take a knife, pierce through the skin into the flesh of the fruit and cut a slit along the length of the banana. Gently open the slit and place the chocolate chunks into the opening. (We've provided no measurements here as you'll have to decide for yourself how much chocolate to use.)

Wrap the banana tightly in the foil and place directly onto the dying coals for about 20 minutes. Carefully remove the foil parcel from the coals and leave to cool for a few minutes. To serve, simply open the foil and eat the flesh from within the skin.

CHOCOLATE BROWNIE CAKE

Meltingly soft, luxuriously rich, this cake is delicious warm or chilled – if you can wait that long to eat it.

Ingredients:

4 eggs

225 g caster sugar

2 drops of vanilla essence

150 g dark chocolate (best if you use 70 per cent cocoa solids)

125 g unsalted butter

50 ml water

25 g plain flour

50 g ground almonds

Preheat oven to 180°C/350°F/gas mark 4. Grease and line an 18 cm springform cake tin.

Break the eggs into a bowl and whisk together with the sugar and vanilla essence until light and fluffy.

Meanwhile, put the chocolate, butter and water in a large bowl and melt together over a bain-marie (place bowl over a pan of simmering water making sure the bowl does not touch the water). Once melted, gently stir all ingredients together with a metal spoon.

Using a metal spoon gently fold the creamed eggs and sugar mixture into the chocolate mix then stir in the flour and almonds.

Pour ingredients into a cake tin and bake for 30–40 minutes until the centre of the torte is still soft, but a thin crust has formed on the surface. Remove from the oven and try not to demolish immediately.

FRUIT CRUMBLE

As desserts go, these have to be one of the most comforting, especially if you serve it with lovely warm custard. The choice of fruit can be anything that suits you and yours.

Apple & blackberry

Ingredients:

For the filling:

3 cooking apples

25 g butter

150 g caster sugar

75 g fresh (or frozen) blackberries

For the crumble:

110 g plain flour

50 g butter, diced

50 g caster sugar

Preheat the oven to 180°C/350°F/ gas mark 4.

Peel, core and slice the apples into equal-sized chunks.

Gently heat the butter in a small pan until melted, then add the apple slices and warm through, until they soften. Add the sugar, and stir well.

Once the sugar has melted, add the blackberries and stir, then remove from the heat.

In a large bowl, sift the flour and add the butter and sugar. Use your fingertips to rub together to create a coarse, breadcrumb texture.

Transfer the filling into an ovenproof dish (approximately 20 cm square). Sprinkle the crumble mixture on top of the filling, making sure you leave no gaps around the sides.

Bake for 20 minutes, or until golden brown.

TOP TIP

It might seem basic but remember a child's stomach is smaller than an adult's so it doesn't need as much food. If they've eaten a decent amount, don't insist they clear their plates as this sort of demand can start to create barriers towards eating, especially if you have a fussy eater.

ETON MESS

This is the easiest dessert to prepare, and it's always a winner.

Ingredients:

450 g soft fruit (strawberries alone or a mix with raspberries, blueberries, etc.)

300 ml whipping or double cream

100 g ready-made meringue

Rinse and hull the strawberries and chop into pieces.

Place the whipping or double cream in a large bowl and whip until light and fluffy. Do not over whip. Break the meringue into bite-sized chunks and gently stir into the cream along with the fruit, avoiding being too brutal – the fruit should keep its shape. Chill in the fridge before spooning into glass bowls to serve.

MICROWAVE APPLE SPONGE

We know not everyone has a microwave, but if you have and want a good tasty pud in minutes, then this one's for you.

Ingredients:

2 large cooking apples

120 g caster sugar

100 g butter

2 eggs

100 g self-raising flour

2 tbsp milk

Peel, core and chop the apples into small chunks and place in a bowl and mix in 20 g of the sugar. Cook the apple for a couple of minutes in the microwave then set aside to cool.

Beat the butter and sugar together in a bowl until it's creamy in colour then beat in the eggs. Sift the flour and fold into the other ingredients until they are fully combined. Add the milk and mix well.

Spoon the cake mixture into the bowl containing the pre-prepared apple then cover with cling film. Microwave on high for 4 minutes until golden brown and springy to the touch.

MICROWAVE SYRUP SPONGE PUDDING

The almost instant results to be had from this microwave recipe will find a soft spot in any child's heart.

Ingredients:

125 g butter, plus extra for basin

2 tbsp syrup

100 g muscovado sugar

2 eggs

125 g self-raising flour

1 tbsp whole milk

Zest of 1 lemon

Grease the insides of a 1 litre microwavable bowl. Spoon in the syrup so that it covers the bottom. In a separate bowl, beat the butter and sugar until smooth. Then add the eggs, one at a time. Add the flour, milk and lemon zest and combine until mixed thoroughly.

Spoon the mixture into the bowl. Cover the bowl with a plate and microwave on full power for 5 minutes. Leave for 3–4 minutes to stand.

Turn out onto a plate and drizzle with more syrup if required. Delicious served with cream or custard.

MILK JELLY

The addition of milk to this traditional party food adds a new dimension and creates great pastel colours.

Ingredients:

1 x 135 g pack of jelly (flavour of your choice)

300 ml water

500 ml whole milk

Break the jelly into cubes and place in a large bowl then pour 300 ml boiling water over and stir until the jelly has completely dissolved. Allow the mixture to cool for about 15–20 minutes or until completely cold, then add the milk. Stir well and pour into a large serving bowl or jelly mould (those old-fashioned ones shaped like rabbits are fun). Chill in the fridge for 2–3 hours or until set.

SIMPLE CHEESECAKE

*There's nothing like a home-made cheesecake and this simple recipe can be
served alone or with any kind of fruit you like.*

Ingredients:

175 g digestive biscuits

75 g butter

150 ml double cream

225 g cream cheese

1 x 175 g tin of condensed milk

Crush the biscuits and mix together
with melted butter then press into a
well-greased 20 cm flan tin/springform
cake tin and chill in a fridge for 10
minutes.

Whip the cream then mix together with
all of the remaining ingredients and
spoon on top of the biscuit mix in the
tin and chill in the fridge for 30 minutes
before serving with fresh fruit.

BREAKFASTS

EGGS

FRIED EGGS ON TOAST

Ingredients:

2 tbsp cooking oil (vegetable or olive)

1 egg per person

Bread for toasting

Butter for spreading on toast

Heat some oil in a frying pan, but don't let the fat get too hot or the egg will stick to the pan and bubble. Crack the egg on the side of the pan and plop the egg into the oil. Fry gently for about 3 minutes, basting occasionally and lifting the edges with a spatula as they cook to prevent sticking. If you like your eggs American-style (over-easy), fry both sides of the egg.

Serve on top of hot, buttered toast.

POACHED EGG

One of the healthiest methods for cooking eggs as it requires no cooking fat or oil.

Ingredients:

1 egg per person

The traditional way of poaching eggs is to boil some water in a saucepan and then, after breaking the egg into a cup or mug, slide it gently into the water. Only put one egg in at a time, and wait for it to firm up before removing with a slotted spoon. An alternative is to use cling film to line a ramekin, crack the egg on top, and then close up the edges of the cling film to create an airtight pouch. You can then put this in the boiling water without fear of your egg breaking and making a gooey mess of your best saucepan.

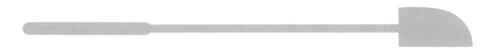

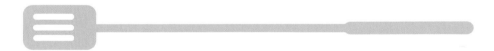

"
As a toddler Sophie was much less fussy than she is today. She would eat almost anything. However recently she is beginning to be more open about trying new things – I put it down to growing up. "

GRAHAM, DAD OF SOPHIE, AGED 6

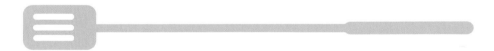

"

I ask Jack to try things that he's said he doesn't like, as well as new foods, by putting a small bit on his plate a couple of times. If, after three or four tries, he still doesn't like it I leave it for a while then try again at a later date. I used to be the world's fussiest eater and have only got better since having Jack. He teaches me as much as I teach him.

"

NIKKI, MUM OF JACK, AGED 8

SCRAMBLED EGG

'Joined up' egg is sometimes more appealing to a child than a separate white and yolk. If you can get your child to enjoy scrambled egg at a young age it's a great way of getting protein into them.

Ingredients:

3 eggs

4 tbsp milk

Seasoning (salt, if desired, and pepper to taste)

25 g butter

Whisk the eggs in a bowl and add the milk and pepper. Melt the butter in a saucepan and add the egg mixture. Stir the mixture continuously as it thickens. Don't have the heat up too high, or else the egg will burn and stick to the pan.

Serve on top of hot, buttered toast.

PANCAKES

Who needs to wait until Shrove Tuesday? This recipe is popular with those who want a cooked breakfast that's not too heavy.

Ingredients:

100 g plain flour

Pinch of salt (if desired)

1 egg

250 ml milk

2 tbsp cooking oil (vegetable or olive) or 50 g butter

Put the flour (and salt if desired) in a bowl and add the egg into the middle. Pour in about a third of the milk. Stir gently, adding the rest of the milk a little at a time. Beat the mixture thoroughly, then pour into a jug.

Melt a small knob of butter in a frying pan or heat a few drops of oil, then add a couple of tablespoons of the batter. Tip the frying pan to spread the mixture evenly. Fry until the underside is brown, using a spatula to lift the edges so that they don't stick, then toss the pancake (or, if there's no one around to impress, you could flip the pancake using a spatula or palette knife).

Tip the finished pancake onto a plate and cover with lemon juice and sugar, then start on the next pancake. Chocolate spread is another popular topping in place of lemon and sugar.

NEVER MiND THe SpROUTS

PORRIDGE

The perfect start to a cold wintry day – nutritious, warming and tasty.

Ingredients:

100 g porridge oats

100 ml milk

300 ml boiling water

Salt (if desired)

Mix the oatmeal and milk into a paste and add boiling water. Heat and simmer in a saucepan for 15 minutes, stirring occasionally. Stir in a pinch of salt if you're using it and serve with syrup, jam or fruit.

SMOOTHIES

BANANA AND RASPBERRY SMOOTHIE

The sometimes sharp flavour of raspberries is offset by the sweetness of the pineapple juice in this wonderfully refreshing smoothie.

Ingredients:

2 bananas

240 ml pineapple juice

120 ml natural yoghurt

175 g raspberries

4 ice cubes

Place all of the ingredients into the blender and blend until smooth.

BREAKFAST SMOOTHIE

This is wonderfully filling and tastes so good you'd be forgiven for forgetting how healthy it actually is.

Ingredients:

1 large banana

200 ml milk

2 tbsp rolled porridge oats

2 tsp runny honey

2 ice cubes

Place all of the ingredients into the blender and blend until smooth.

KIWI AND MELON SMOOTHIE

Zingy and sweet, super-healthy and refreshing – the perfect smoothie!

Ingredients:

½ honeydew melon

1 kiwi fruit

1 apple

2 tsp honey

4 ice cubes

Peel and slice the melon and kiwi fruit. Peel the apple and core it, then cut into small chunks. Place all of the ingredients into the blender and blend until smooth.

MANGO, STRAWBERRY AND BANANA SMOOTHIE

Try adding a sprinkling of rolled oats or muesli on top to make this a more substantial breakfast.

Ingredients:

5 strawberries

100 g mango flesh

1 small banana

200 ml apple juice

Wash the strawberries carefully and cut off the green leafy tops. Peel and chop the mango. Place all of the ingredients into the blender and blend until smooth.

STRAWBERRY SMOOTHIE

Perfect for those who prefer a lighter start to the day. You could try experimenting with different fruits and juices – use whatever is in season to save the planet as well as your pennies.

Ingredients:

½ cantaloupe melon

10 strawberries

240 ml orange juice

4 ice cubes

Peel the melon, remove the seeds and cube the flesh. Wash the strawberries thoroughly and cut off the green leafy tops. Place all of the ingredients into the blender and blend until smooth.

INDEX

SPROUTS QUESTIONNAIRE RESULTS

MOST FAVOURED FOODS:

Pasta

Pizza

Chips

Wraps

Roast potatoes

Mild curry

Sausages

Chicken

Cheese

Carrots

Cucumber

Strawberries

Apples

Grapes

Rice

Tomatoes

Broccoli

Ham

MOST DISLIKED FOODS:

Casserole (meat)

Cheese

Mash

Shepherd's pie

Red meat, especially fatty or gristly meat

Mince

Onions

Potatoes

Tomatoes (raw)

WHAT IMPACTS CHOICE THE MOST?

Texture

Smell

Taste

Appearance is not usually a deciding factor.

HAVE YOU TRIED TO CHANGE YOUR CHILD'S EATING HABITS?

Exactly half of those who completed the questionnaire had tried to change their child's eating habits, the remaining half had not.

FOODS MOST DISLIKED BY ADULTS:

Cabbage, sprouts, cauliflower: taste

Fish: smell/texture

Offal (kidney, liver, heart): smell

NOTES

....
....
....
....
....
....
....
....
....
....
....
....
....
....
....
....
....
....
....

NEVER MiND THe SpROUTS

If you're interested in finding out more about our books,
find us on Facebook at **Summersdale Publishers** and
follow us on Twitter at **@Summersdale**.

www.summersdale.com